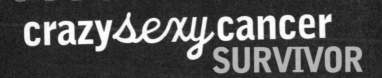

crazy*sexy* cancer
SURVIVOR

More Rebellion and Fire for Your Healing Journey

kris carr

foreword by
MARIANNE WILLIAMSON

skirt!®

Guilford, Connecticut
An imprint of The Globe Pequot Press

The health information expressed in this book is based solely on the personal experience of the author and is not intended as a medical manual. The information should not be used for diagnosis or treatment, or as a substitute for professional medical care. The author and publisher urge you to consult with your health care provider prior to attempting any treatment on yourself or another individual.

skirt!® is an attitude . . . spirited, independent, outspoken, serious, playful and irreverent, sometimes controversial, always passionate.

Photo credits: spot art throughout provided by ClipArt.com and CSA Images; p. viii by Paul Bednarski; p. 18 by Eric Stephen Jacobs; p. 29 © photos.com; p. 39 courtesy Julie Larson; p. 77 courtesy Terri Cole; p. 88 by Bill Frakes courtesy Ginger Southall; p. 159 courtesy Ann Orcutt; p. 174 courtesy Beth Villandry; pp. 218 and 229 by Mark Morford courtesy Sera Beak. All other photographs courtesy Kris Carr.

Design by Karla Baker: www.typekarla.com

Library of Congress Cataloging-in-Publication Data
Carr, Kris.
  Crazy sexy cancer survivor : more rebellion and fire for your healing journey / Kris Carr ; foreword by Marianne Williamson.
     p. cm.
  ISBN 978-1-59921-370-5
  1. Cancer in women—Popular works. I. Title.
  RC281.W65C3738 2008
  616.99'40082—dc22

                                        2008006047

Printed in the United States of America
10 9 8 7 6 5 4 3 2 1

For my teacher, friend, confidante,
and spiritual daughter Crystal
(like the expensive champagne).
Thank you for the unconditional love
and sweet purrs.

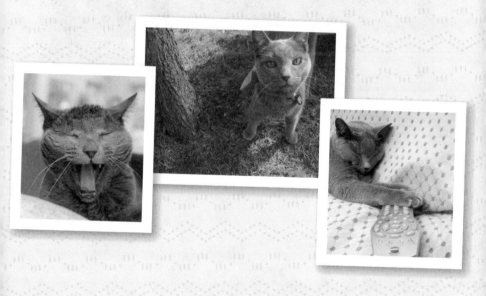

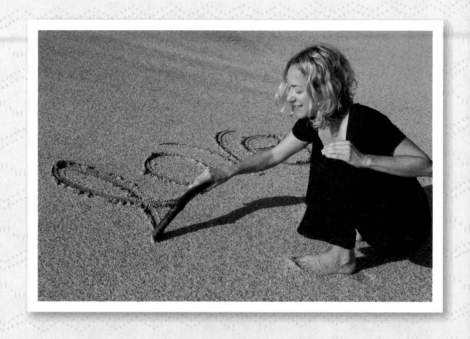

A survivor is a triumphant person who lives with, after, or in spite of a diagnosis or traumatic event. Survivors refuse to assume the identity of their adversity. They are not imprisoned by the constructs of a label. Instead, survivors use their brush with mortality as a catalyst for creating a better self. We transform our experience in order to further evolve spiritually, emotionally, physically, and mentally. Our reality challenges us to go deeper.

Survivors cultivate an essence that will never be victim to a word.

(inspired by Beth Villandry)

contents

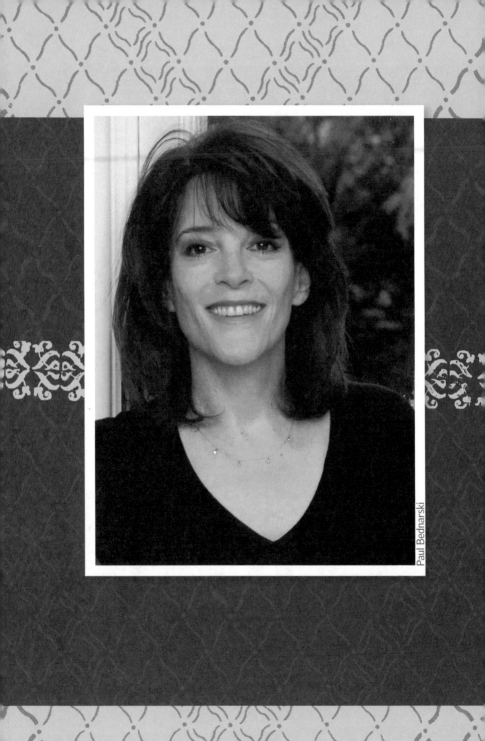

foreword

I met Kris when I saw her introduce her film *Crazy Sexy Cancer* at the Urban Zen holistic conference in New York City. When Kris spoke, you could hear a pin drop. She told her tale of coming to terms with a diagnosis of a rare, incurable cancer—a devastating blow to anyone, but especially to a young person. Yet her story—told with grace and humor as well as a beautiful, empowering embrace of every person in the audience—was a message not of devastation but of triumph. One felt from her only the most palpable celebration of life, and a profound ability to turn a horrific challenge into a quest for personal transformation.

WITH THE MOVIE AND HER BOOK *CRAZY SEXY CANCER TIPS*, I THINK KRIS HAS BEGUN A REVOLUTION.

Cancer having become the health epidemic of our time, people are looking for psychological, emotional, nutritional, and spiritual advice as much as they are looking for medical advice. Kris has already given hope to thousands of people—particularly young adults who are dealing with this often heartbreaking challenge—and I predict that she will ultimately bring hope and comfort to millions.

Kris has toured the country sharing her message, and in short order has become a fresh, authentic, empowering voice. I recommend Kris to you in the highest possible terms. She is an inspirational speaker and original thinker, with a message that puts cancer firmly in its place. She presents a path, clearly paved by her own grit and tears, by which others can move forward out of despair and into hope. I say *Bravo* to her from the bottom of my heart. She is simply gorgeous, inside and out.

Marianne Williamson

introduction:

LET DESPERATION LEAD TO
inspiration and education

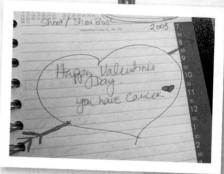

My universal smackdown came on Valentine's Day 2003, when I had what I call my needle-off-the-record moment: "You have cancer." Those words will forever be tattooed on my soul. Thursday, I was an aspiring young actress and photographer living in New York City. By Friday at 2 p.m.—*BAM*—I was a cancer patient.

As I wrote in my first book, I'd thought I just had a hangover, but when my Jivamukti yoga class didn't provide its usual kick-ass cure, a visit to my doctor revealed that my liver was covered with lesions. That wasn't all, though; *non, non, mon cherie*. The tumors had spread to my lungs. And get this: The cancer was completely inoperable, with no cure and no definitive treatment.

The good news was that the cancer appeared to be a slow-moving sarcoma, epithelioid hemangioendothelioma to be exact. Huh? I could barely pronounce it, let alone come to grips with the fact that it was growing inside me. Sarcomas are cancers that affect the soft tissues, nerves, muscles, joints, and bones. They're extremely rare and mysterious, and because so few patients are diagnosed with them, research funds aren't exactly overflowing. This is why sarcomas are often called "the forgotten cancer." Still, because of its unique genetic makeup, my cancer wasn't behaving aggressively. So in one sense I had what every cancer patient longs for: time.

The bad news was that this could change at any moment. My only option was to take a watch-and-wait, learn-to-live-with-cancer approach. Wow, please dump me into a bottomless vat of scotch!

Learn to live with a Stage IV cancer? How? How could I learn to live with cancer without thinking of dying every day? That's when the lightbulb blazed on. To move through the fear, I had to change my focus and turn to the one thing that had always saved me in hard times: creativity.

Within weeks I had picked up my camera and my pen and begun documenting my story. *Crazy Sexy Cancer*, I called it. Why not? If I had to live with this beastie, I didn't want to shrivel, hide, or feel like damaged goods. I needed to hoot and holler. The title freed me to feel normal and giggle again while the creative project gave me something productive and tangible to anchor my future to. The result is my documentary film as well as my first book, *Crazy Sexy Cancer Tips*, a righteous guide to kicking cancer tail.

Cancer Is a Guru

Let's just say it like it is: Cancer creates pandemonium. Your life is forever changed and there will always be a virginity stolen by cancer. Yet so many people who've been through it swear it was the best thing that ever happened to them. Why? Because if you let it, cancer will take you to your zero point and teach you how to live like you mean it. We are all warriors, angels, and stunning revolutionaries—cancer can't take that away from us. I would rather hemorrhage in a pool of starving sharks than let cancer break my spirit or make me feel like a sick person. So I *choose* to believe that I am more alive, more beautiful, and, yes, sexier (aka more empowered, passionate, and intriguing) than ever before! Why not? Cancer is nothing to be ashamed of. You didn't fail. I understand feeling angry and powerless in the wake of this disease all too well. But aren't we all so tired of swallowing the pain and suffering and fearing words we dare not say?

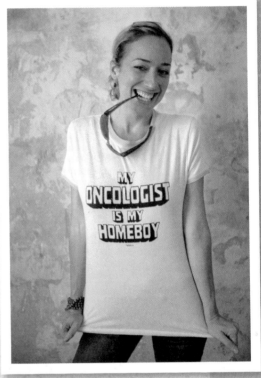

What if you could shift your perception and come to understand the big C (or any major challenge in your life) not as the stereotypical death sentence but as a *chance*—to learn, to dive deep, to grow and smash stigmas, to truly *live life.* What if you could see adversity as an adventure instead of a battle, an opportunity and not a curse? The big-daddy life question isn't whether we're going to die. I got news for ya, life is a terminal condition; cancer patients are just more aware of it. The real question is how many of us will choose to truly live. No one will give you license to carpe diem. You are the only one who can make the decision to go for it. If you're reading this, you probably got the big wake-up call. Are you going to let it go to voice mail—once again?

There is a wealth of tips, tricks, and insights available to help you navigate the labyrinth that is cancer. Let this book show you how to slide into the driver's seat and turn on your internal GPS. Your wisdom goes far beyond these pages. Each of us can tap into the ancient voodoo chili sage that intuitively knows what to do and which direction to shimmy. If you hush the chatter for a second, you'll hear it. Perhaps it will sound like a whisper—or maybe it'll blow out your eardrums with the stadium rumble of a Springsteen concert.

See the Angel and Set Her Free

When I excavated my internal compass, I began to understand what the master sculptor, painter, and architect Michelangelo meant when he described how he "released" the brilliant (not to mention hot) statue *David:* "I saw the angel in the marble and carved until I set him free." Michelangelo had the genius to see the masterpiece inside a big rock. Then with focus, commitment, and follow-through, he brought his vision to life.

There's a work of art inside you, too, buried beneath fear, doubt, and untapped wildfire. Everything you need lies dormant in your heart. This workbook will give you the tools to excavate that ruby and let your inner goddess shine! Get messy, dig around, be truthful, and call yourself out: What's the frickin' game plan, yo? Roll up your sleeves and have a come-to-JBEE (Jesus, Buddha, Elvis, Etc.) session. I like to sit with my journal, spill the beans, wipe up the mess, reframe, and refocus. If you let it, this book can help you shake off the passive malaise and set you on the path toward deep healing. Think of it as your private sacred space, a creative wall to throw some spelt spaghetti on. And just because I call it a workbook doesn't mean it's a study hall drag. Have fun with these pages! Doodle, babble, bleed, rant, and play. Dream big but leave room for magic.

Light a Candle

High-roller trauma can light a burning inner fire. It shakes us from our monochrome box of perceptions and soaks our world in Technicolor. Cancer teaches us to ride our fear even though it bucks like

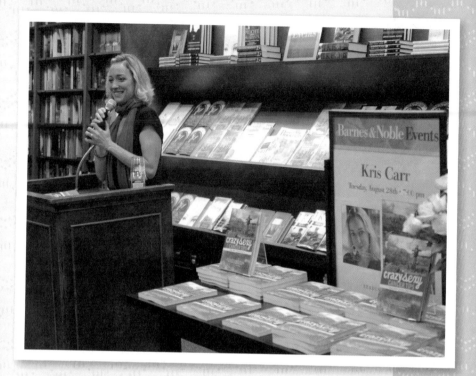

a mechanical dragon. If we resist the bucking, it will
be a very bumpy ride and more than likely we'll fall.
But if we go with the rhythm and flow, we can ride
that dragon forever. The choice is ours. As my pistol-
packin' granny used to say: *Don't curse the darkness, light a candle.*

The darkness is a call to action, and your freedom
lies in taking the first step. Don't worry about the
entire staircase, just take one step, and then tomor-
row take another.

Firestarter

I get lots of awesome letters from people around the
world. As I've dropped my walls and shared my story
with honesty (and a dash of naughty humor), it has
encouraged others to do the same. I used to pry open
doors just wide enough to get my toes slammed in
them. Success was something I longed for but rarely

experienced in a sustainable way. Yet since the Crazy Sexy revolution started, doors have been flying off the hinges. I have had the privilege of shaking thousands of hands, have helped raise lots of moolah for different cancer organizations, and turned doctors into colleagues and medicine men into pen pals.

Heck, I even got to chat 'n' chew with the queen herself, Ms. Oprah Winfrey. *"Oprah, I'm coming, save me a seat!"* I used to write in my journal as I worked on my projects, especially when I had my doubts. *Note:* Manifestation has major mojo! And now here I was pinching myself till my arm turned black and blue as I sat on her stage talking about love, death, veggies, and ass-kickin' strategies for living the best life ever. All while glancing into the loving eyes of the man in the front row, my husband, Brian. As I dished in my first book, cancer was my matchmaker. I share all of this to prove that life doesn't stop when the turbulent ouchies come. In some cases, if you can get through the bumps, you'll unwrap abundantly sweet fruit baskets.

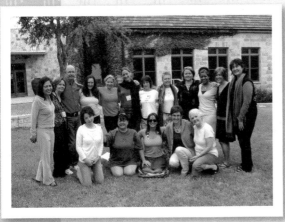

The first Crazy Sexy Cancer boot camp, Austin 2008

Join the celebration (http://my.crazy sexylife.com). If you haven't read the first book, I encourage you to do so. Crazy Sexy fans are an outrageous bunch! They stomp with sparks and grace. They push boundaries and never take no for an answer. To Crazy Sexies *no* means *go!* Oodles of cowgirls and dudes with all kinds of experiences (not just cancer) have hopped on the bandwagon. There is a community, a global wellness posse forming as you read this sentence. Why? Because the Crazy Sexy attitude taps into

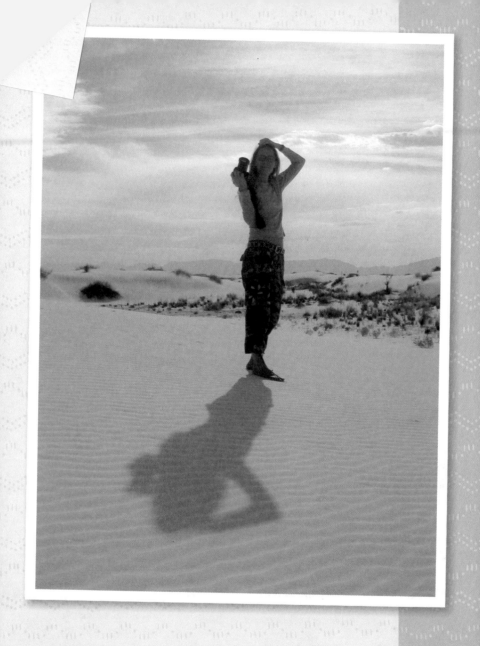

life's sweet spot, the place in each of us where possibility meets human potential. Where curiosity hugs *Why not?*

This time around I will introduce you to a posse of wellness professionals, a few friends, and two cherished power women in my family. I have found deep value in creating my own support community, and I urge you to do the same. *Crazy Sexy Cancer Survivor* is broken down into four parts: diagnosis, mind, body, and spirit. Each offers reflections and suggestions for the ride. A few of the stories you'll remember from *Crazy Sexy Cancer Tips*—nuggets so delicious it wouldn't hurt you to taste them again.

You don't have to be a canSer patient (misspelled to bring the oxygen back into the room) to benefit from this workbook. This book is a firestarter, an inner-revolution boot camp. It is full of stories, exercises, meditations, "aha" moments, excavations, rituals, and midnight-ramble-back-porch brainstorms—for everyone. It's meant to inspire you to become an empowered participant in your healing. This isn't about canSer, this is about life, and *life* is a juggernaut of gorgeous, staggering, messy, brilliant, *yes, no,* holy cow, holy shit, champagne supernova, love, loss, and learning. The only thing you have to bring to this is a willingness to be fearless. No one gets an easy pass; we're all hauling around something, and we can either drown in the suffering or use it as a springboard for personal metamorphosis. Our spunky attitude is the key to our freedom. So what are you going to do? Wither on the vine or bloom, beauty, bloom? Open up, breathe in, and let yourself *thrive!*

Turn the page. I dare you.

PART ONE:
diagnosis 101

WHAT TO EXPECT
WHEN YOU ARE NOT EXPECTING
. . . A DIAGNOSIS

Okay, Cowgirl and dude: Stay calm. Anyone who has been diagnosed with the pesky big C knows that it's a crisis of the mind as well as the body. We immediately imagine the worst and bust our knees praying for a kind yet authoritative soul to tell us that this nightmare is all a heinous mistake. But no one ever does. Instead we are abruptly introduced to our mortality. *"Greetings, Death. I'm [insert name] and I'm not ready for you yet so BACK OFF!"* Time stops as the perception of safety and freedom slowly vanishes and suddenly we deeply understand that dorky old saying, "Without our health, we have nothing."

In this section we'll revisit some basic strategies for creating a solid foundation from which healing can flourish. By addressing potential practical and emotional road blocks and learning how to overcome them, you will be reminded of your personal power in every given moment and the importance of having compassion both for yourself and for your kickin' crew. Digest the precious lessons hidden among the terror and statistics and focus on building a better you.

Cancer demands that we get off our asses and *GO FOR IT*—I mean, what are we waiting for? Out with the complaints, in with the solutions. Give yourself a tune up from the inside out. As you grow and change, so will your maintenance plan. Make a pact with yourself to continually survey your inner landscape and upgrade your lifestyle accordingly.

It's your turn.
Renovate and read on.

Good morning sunshine, you are a Survivor!

If you haven't already, now is the time to give yourself authorization to define your own journey. Put yourself in a can-do space. In my mind, you are a survivor the day you are diagnosed. As women and men with cancer we live every day with a suffocating weight on our throats. *What if? Will I see my next birthday? Can I get married? If so, can I have children?* Perhaps you've already fashioned your nest, yet in less grounded moments you find yourself paralyzed with angst, imagining yourself gone and your kids being raised by a stripper. CanSer (or any adversity) puts us on the rim and while we are on the rim we have an opportunity to appreciate and express fear simultaneously. We multitask dying with living while managing our chores in order to keep it together and stay out of prison. So why not celebrate all that we've managed to accomplish already? Sometimes just keeping it together is surviving.

Don't be timid or feel like you are jinxing yourself. Stand up straight and yodel the S word! Survivors come in many shapes and sizes. The best part about being a survivor is the appreciation we feel for the little things (even when they're painful): the sheer joy of peeing in the ocean; of crying so hard that you burst into giggle madness; the agony of suffering over a lost love or a perished dream. Survivors squeeze every drop of delicious juice from this extraordinary life.

From diagnosis to discovery, survivor is an attitude. You, my friend, are a survivor no matter what. I am a survivor. We don't wait 'til the icy patch thaws before celebrating life. We see freedom, create it, become it. When I put cancer behind me and started smiling again, the disease lost its grip on me. Isn't that what the "cure" is all about?

Write it here . . . I am a SURVIVOR, a Crazy Sexy Survivor and thriver! Now twirl!

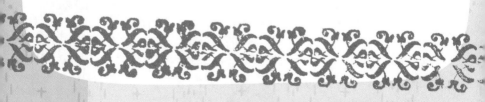

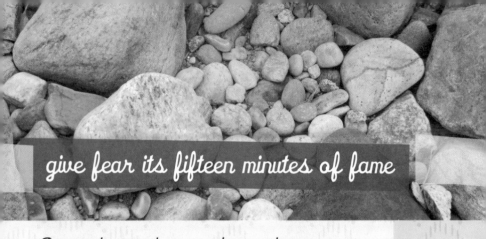

give fear its fifteen minutes of fame

Fear can be more dangerous than any disease. It swipes our joy and tramples our hope. Days, weeks, even years can slip through your fingers. If left unchecked, fear will strangle every breath from our lives. I am constantly amazed by the many paradoxes in this gorgeous life. Why is it that we're so scared to live and yet so afraid to die? We thirst for change and yet we choose to remain stuck. Trippy, right? How many of us dwell in that self-imposed purgatory? I know I've spent a good portion of my young life loping around and marking time, treating life as if it were a dress rehearsal and I was the understudy.

The first step in taking charge of your situation is to acknowledge the fear. Let it have its fifteen minutes (or more) of fame. What are you afraid of? Many of our fears are totally justified and need to be heard before they can be soothed. Those are healthy fears. Unhealthy fears are the ones that are purely negative and spread like an itchy VD. Those are the ones that need some TLC and a dab of cream!

Do a reality scan and have a come-to-JBEE (Jesus, Buddha, Elvis, Etc.) moment with yourself. Feel your body, hear your breath, ground yourself in the right now. Ask yourself if your fears are manageable or if they determine your every thought, word, and action. Allow the honest answer to come forward. If the response is a booming, "Yes, they rule my life," then inner chaos is bound to clog you up. Few things are worse than soul constipation. It hurts and makes you feel cranky and fat.

What are you afraid of?

Write it down. Once you put your fears on paper, here's a hot idea: **BURN THEM!** Put the bastards in a cauldron and release them from your life. Dance naked if ya like.

NOW RIP THIS PAGE OUT AND BURN IT!

Snap Out of It!

The peace and calm of a collected mind can be yours, but it takes time and work. The doctor can't prescribe a pill to make the terror go away, and Suzanne Somers won't sell you serenity on QVC. Dial it down a notch and breathe. Throughout the day, stop yourself every time you get that belly surge—you know, the one that surfs your lunch back up on a wave of panic. Count to ten. On the inhale count one; on the exhale count one. Inhale two, exhale two, and so on.

Breathing and Visualization

Attaching a visual to your breathing increases your ability to regain control. Here's an image that works for me: As I inhale I visualize golden sunlight warming and filling my body. The light is divine, it illuminates my corners and releases stored tension. As I exhale I imagine the darkness pouring out of my body like dirty water. This exercise is cleansing for me, a rebirth. My grime is absorbed into the ground as my body is rejuvenated by the healing God energy of the sun. What resonates with you? When we practice visualization on a regular basis we strengthen our ability to manage fear and pain.

Panic jump-starts those little party hats that sit on top of your kidneys known as adrenals. Back in the day when we were chased by lions, our adrenals encouraged us to *run!* Now they short-circuit dozens of times per day thanks to our stressful modern world. Add cancer to the stew, and your nerves are shot. Fight-or-flight hormones course through your system at dangerous levels on a regular basis. I don't have to be a doctor to tell you it's unhealthy to live in that space. How do you stop, drop, and roll? My posse gal Terri Cole uses an interesting technique. Check this out . . .

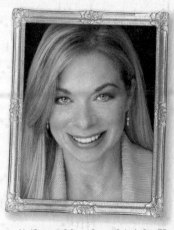

As a life coach and psychotherapist, a big part of my job is to help people make changes in their lives. I have found a very effective tool for stopping self-sabotaging behavior, whether it be weight loss, drug or alcohol addiction, or compulsive thoughts. I call it the rubber band trick. You place a loose rubber band around your wrist, and as soon as you are aware of a negative thought—a plan to eat the doughnut, drink the booze, meet up with X dealer, or arrange your funeral—you snap the rubber band and think *stop*. In therapeutic circles it is known as aversion therapy, and it's a variation on cognitive behavioral therapy (CBT).

Although CBT is typically used to treat anxiety, depression, and other mental conditions, by adding a simple twist it can be used to break thought patterns and behaviors that don't serve us. During my cancer experience and subsequent treatment, when I found myself falling into the scary what-ifs, I used this rubber band technique to stop the negative thought pattern and to shock my body and mind back to the present moment. The realization that I had the power to change my thoughts made me feel empowered and took the edge off my fear.

As human beings, we are wired to avoid pain. So once you associate negative scary thoughts or behavior with the mild pain of snapping the rubber band, gradually the behavior or thought pattern will dissipate, leaving you more brain space, time, and energy to focus on the much more important business of healing wonderful you.

1

2

3

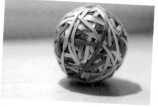

Stuffed Emotions

There are no hard-and-fast rules on how to deal with a diagnosis. I wish I could give you a road map, but I can't. When you're newly diagnosed, everyone who loves you wigs out, not just you. Friendships shift (or tank). Family roles and dynamics change, sometimes forever. But you are not cancer.

Physical setbacks and hardship kick up a lot of stored emotions. Oftentimes these emotions, especially compacted anger, can slow down the healing process. Letting out the gunky junk might make you feel out of control, as if once the looting gremlins are out of the box all hell will break loose. Remember, feelings aren't facts. Feelings are signposts. Read them and navigate accordingly (wear your seatbelt too, as it may be a turbulent ride).

Really listen to the whispers or bellows of your body. What are they telling you? Locate the area in your temple that feels neglected or isolated. Give that part a voice, a way to communicate with you. For example, when I do this exercise I imagine the quadruple six-pack of tumors that currently reside in my liver and lungs and I chat with them. Notice I said "currently reside." I view the little suckers as temporary tutors, not permanent parasites. My tutors have a unique voice; they actually sound like Smurfs. Our periodic summit meetings clear the air and give us active marching orders. Here's what they've said in the past: "I'm steaming mad!" *At who?* I say, *About what, darling?* Whoa you'd be surprised what vomits up and out. Let your Smurfs vent. They'll feel better and so will you; because the healthiest way to dissolve the pain is to stare it in the eye and dance with it. See your truth, hear your truth, transform your truth. Resisting pain is like arm wrestling with a two-year-old. Your pain will fuss and freak and you will never truly win.

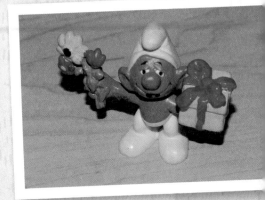

When we tighten from trauma, our energetic flow is constricted. Are there areas of your body that resist the glow? If so, spend a few minutes and consciously turn your attention inward. Take a deep breath and gaze upon the puss. What does it look like? If your body were a billboard, what would it say? Did you need to hit a wall in order to redirect your life? As you know, I'm not a mystic or a social worker; these are just some of the questions I've asked myself at various pit stops on my trip.

Now you ask. Start by looking inside your beautiful God pod and read that inner billboard.
Draw it.
Consider using crayons and stickers.

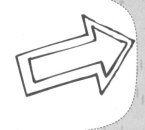

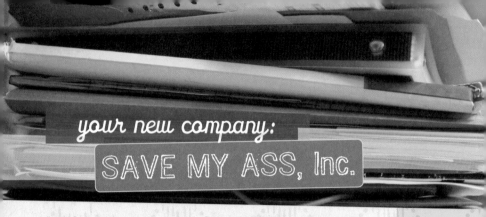

While juggling your already busy life, you've suddenly been catapulted into the "biohazardous" world of cancer. Critical decisions await, and I encourage you to find the
strength to spearhead your strategy. You and you alone are
responsible for your health. You are the boss, the CEO. You
are in charge, and no one knows more about your body than
you do! The key to success is to handpick a staff of winners
to work by your side. Doctors, nurses, healers, alternative
health practitioners, family, friends, and helpers are all vital
members of your workforce.

WHEN YOU HIRE A DOCTOR, IMAGINE THAT THERE'S A JOB OPEN AT YOUR COMPANY.

If the applicant isn't a perfect match, "No hard feelings and thanks for your time but I need someone more
qualified." Remember, *she* works for *you!* Don't try to jam
a square peg into a round hole. Move on, and when I say
move I mean *travel.* Do not be lazy or go limp. If the doctor
you choose doesn't have her finger on the pulse of the latest
research, then get in the car and go. You don't owe anyone
anything!

Crazy Sexy Beth MD

Open yourself up to the precious people you'll meet along the cancer trail. A tall glass of bubbly came bouncing my way in my new friend Beth. We met after a lecture I gave in New York City, and my life has been blessed ever since. Beth shoots from the hip and has a heart as big as the Grand Canyon. She is a doctor and a CanSer Cowgirl, so she stands on both sides of the white coat. Her presence on my blog (http://crazysexycancer.blogspot.com—join us!) is so big that we nicknamed her Crazy Sexy Beth MD and welcome her regular contribution of tough love, sound advice, and sparkles. Here's Beth's remarkable story . . .

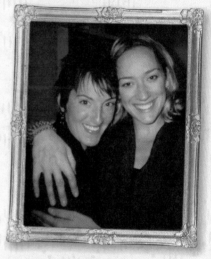

Thanksgiving Day, 2005. I didn't go to my parents' house for dinner, I was sick, had been all week. As a medical resident, it wasn't unusual to pick up whatever virus was floating around the hospital, so I didn't think too much of it. However, by day's end, I had been admitted to the hospital with suspected meningitis. By week's end, after a "visit" from the Code Team, I landed in the intensive care unit. What the heck was going on? This clearly wasn't meningitis. I had no clue, but based on how tight my sphincter felt, I knew it was an *oh shit!* situation.

I spent the next two months in that hospital. Lots of tests, all repeated several times, indicated a problem. But everything about my case was so "unusual," "atypical," that no one could quite put the pieces together. Based on blood tests, my providers thought I had a tumor. I lost track of how many imaging studies I had; truth be told, most of that time was a blur. Long story short, they were unable to locate the tumor.

Things started to turn ugly. No picture of the tumor . . . so it must not exist, right? Many of my care providers—people I know and work with—began to doubt there was anything wrong with me (other than my head). Some stopped returning the nurse's pages. I was yelled at to get out of the hospital. (Yet I couldn't sit up in bed for very long without passing out. Forget about standing up.) The accusations started to fly. I must be doing something to make myself sick. I must be secretly snorting cocaine in my hospital room. I *must* be faking the lab data in the computer somehow. Right?

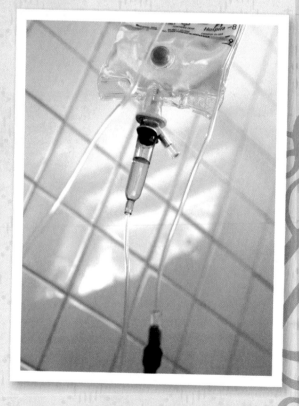

Wrong! But what do you do when, as a patient, your health care team not only stops taking care of you, but effectively abandons you? More than once I was put in the position of having to treat myself when my vital signs were at dangerous limits. When you are in that hospital bed, you are really at the mercy of your team. Nothing happens unless they make it happen. Otherwise you continue to just sit there. The pressure to discharge me was getting ugly. And I was terrified at the thought of what would happen to me if they did.

I knew there was something terribly wrong. I knew I was not getting the comprehensive care I required. Luckily, I also knew how to navigate the health care system. I got on the phone, called mentors, colleagues, friends. I got the name and number of a doctor in a nearby state, and I insisted I be moved to a Boston hospital under his care. For once, in the face of so many naysayers, I stood up and advocated for myself, my care, my health. And it is likely the only reason I am alive today. Turns out, I had a plum-size tumor in my heart. Needless to say, I wasn't faking it. One more month in that Boston hospital, and I came out one mammajammer (that's my friends' name for the tumor) lighter.

I have lots of mixed emotions about that initial part of my canSer trail ride. But the key for all you other CanSer Cowgirls and dudes is to trust yourself. Speak up for what you know to be true. Don't let your doctors make you doubt yourself, your own body, your instincts. And if they've stopped listening, find someone who will. It might just save your life, too.

It's time to **TAKE YOUR DOCTOR'S PULSE**.
How's your relationship going?

List the **three things you like most about her**:

1 ....

....

....

....

2 ....

....

....

....

3 ....

....

....

....

....

List the **three things that most drive you batty:**

1

2

3

If you could design your **DREAM DOCTOR**, what would he look like?

....

....

....

....

....

....

....

....

How does he match up with your real-world version?

....

....

....

....

....

....

....

....

....

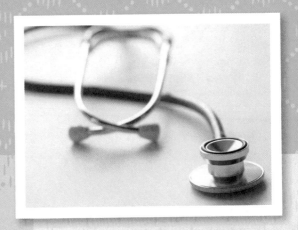

You and Your Doctor, by Crazy Sexy Beth MD

You have an incredible amount of power in the relationship between you and your physician. For some reason, people get in front of a white coat and throw their own instincts, knowledge, and decision-making capabilities out the window. Hell, I've done it, too, and I have a white coat of my own! So what can you do to empower yourself to make this relationship successful?

First and foremost, this is a relationship—ideally a partnership—that like any other relationship will have aspects that work seamlessly, and others that need a bit of cultivating. Doctors are not the enemy. Contrary to popular opinion, they are not responsible for the state of our health care system. That problem is way more complex than simply blaming the providers. So let's see what we can do in our half of the relationship to make it work.

tip 1:

Do unto your doctor . . . Enter into your relationship with your doctor with a positive, embracing attitude—not one of anger, defensiveness, or mistrust. Hostility is a bad note on which to start any relationship. This can be hard, especially if you've had bad experiences. But just like every man isn't that horrible boyfriend who cheated on you, every doctor is not the bad guy who came before. If his actions merit a smackdown—well, that's another story. But don't assume this from the get-go. Project the attitude with which you want to be treated. Okay, maybe a little golden-rulish, but ain't it the truth? Start the relationship off with the right attitude, with a clean slate, moving forward, not looking back.

tip 2:

Set priorities. Define for yourself, when selecting a doctor, what your priorities are. Do you need/ want a doctor who is going to have all kinds of charm? Or is it more important to you that she be immersed in the study, research, and treatment of your disease? Personally, I am willing to sacrifice some of the charm for a doc whom I know can go commando on my cancer, because she knows it from every angle. I can get the warm fuzzies from friends, family, social workers, shrinks, and so on. But that's me. Lots of other people need to feel a connection with their care provider to develop that working relationship. Which is completely understandable. There is no right or wrong way here, folks. Just be clear on what you need from the dynamic.

tip 3:

Clarify your expectations—then communicate them to your doctor. Do you expect your physician to personally call you with results? Within what time frame do you want to hear something? Do you expect your doctor to be available weekends? Holidays? If not, how are those times covered? If you are hospitalized, do you expect your doctor to come in to see you that day? Much of this has to do with the workings of the health care system, but not understanding these things up front leads to a lot of patients getting upset. Sit down in a quiet space with pen and paper and make a list of every conceivable question, scenario, or problem you could have. You might be surprised that a big list will break down to be a few core procedural questions. Then discuss these with your doctor.

tip 4:

Be picky. You are *not* stuck with the first doctor you see. If the vibe between you two is just not happening, or if he's too far toward the Attila-the-Hun extreme with his bedside manner, go see someone else! Kris said it oh so clearly: *You* employ *him*, not the other way around. Do not be afraid to say, "Thank you, but no thank you." In my opinion (and yes, I am probably biased), your doctor is really your right-hand person in your canSer challenge. This needs to be someone you can work with long-term. Don't sweat the bumps in the road; you may have an off interaction once or twice, as in any relationship. Keep it in perspective. Select your doctor just as carefully as you would select a mate, because this is a "life partnership" as well . . . . *your* life.

tip 5:

Be prepared. Before your visit, write down a list of questions, in order of importance to you. Be reasonable about the length of your list. Your doctor is operating under time constraints that are *not* self-imposed (hello, insurance companies). He'd love nothing more than to go over everything with you, but he can't always do that in one visit. Depending on the complexity of your questions, it is reasonable to expect your top five to get answered that day. If you have some still on the list, discuss with your doc how these will get addressed. Can you come back for a fifteen-minute appointment the following week? Can he review them later and e-mail you the responses?

Can a nurse or physician's assistant field some of the questions? You can also hang on to them and bring them to the next appointment. Your provider may be able to get to all of them. But if he can't, it doesn't mean he doesn't want to or isn't interested. Work with him, and I guarantee he'll not only answer all your questions but often go above and beyond in getting information to you.

tip 6:

Be prompt. Don't you hate having to wait for the doctor if she's running late? I know I do. So please, hold up your end of the bargain . . . be on time for your visit! And that doesn't mean showing up at the precise moment of your appointment. It means showing up fifteen minutes beforehand to check in, get any paperwork or insurance info updated or completed, get your vital signs taken, complete blood work, and so on. Doctors—again thanks to good ol' Mr. Insurance—have appointments scheduled back-to-back from the minute they get there until the end of the day, often with few or no breaks. If you, as an early-morning appointment, are even ten minutes late, that throws off the whole day (because many appointments are scheduled in fifteen-minute intervals). Toss in the inevitable emergency and the schedule goes, well, you know where. Believe me, your doctor dislikes running late just as much as you do, if not more. Do your part to keep the day moving; don't be late for your very important date!

tip 7:

Boundaries. Set your boundaries with your doctor at visit number one. Who is your provider allowed to give information to? How do you want to be contacted—e-mail, phone? Do you want a message left? Discuss the specifics of a possible hospitalization. Who will be caring for you? A resident service? One of your physician's partners? Hospitalists? Are you okay with all that? Do you know from the get-go that there are treatments or interventions you *don't* want? Set your boundaries. This *helps* your doctor, so don't feel shy, demanding, or any other negative thing. Believe it or not, most doctors really just want to take the best care of you possible. But they need to know what that means for you, 'cause everyone is different.

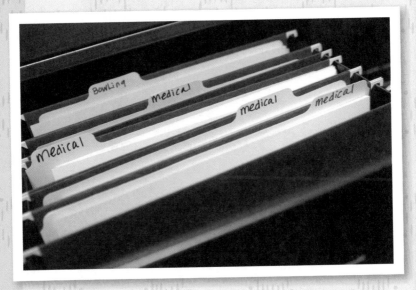

tip 8:

Paperwork. Have your Living Will, advance directives, and health care proxy paperwork completed, signed, and notarized if needed. Everyone, big, small, healthy, or otherwise should have this paperwork done. It's standard practice for providers to ask patients about this paperwork when they are admitted, regardless of their diagnosis. It is not a suggestion that you are dying, or even heading in that direction. It is simply asking you to make sure your wishes are clear so that, God forbid, if the poop ever hits the fan for any reason, things are being handled as you would want them to be. Discuss this with your family. If they are not on board with your choices, they can sometimes be a kink in the process (in other words, change your plans). So communicate, when things are calm and quiet.

I learned this one the hard way . . . I didn't have all this paperwork done myself. I know, mea culpa, mea culpa. But then, there I was in the hospital, being told I might not make it off that operating table, and I was scrambling to get my affairs in order. Not a good time to do this. It is an emotional, upsetting, exhausting enough time without also having to try to find the clarity to make decisions about end-of-life care. You may find yourself choosing things you otherwise wouldn't if the situation weren't so emotionally charged. So do it now, when you are stable, when you can be clear about your wishes. If you don't understand what terms such as *being resuscitated, DNR,* and *DNI* (do not intubate) mean, *ask.* You can't make informed decisions if you don't understand what each entails. Again, involve your family; you want everyone on the same page.

tip 9:

Be honest about what meds you are taking, what other treatments you might be utilizing, and your lifestyle choices. Doctors don't ask these questions to be judge and jury; they just can't be as effective without all the information. This may seem like a ridiculous tip—a no-brainer, right? Well, you might be surprised to learn that most patients underreport. Include any over-the-counter meds you are taking as well as herbal supplements and vitamins. Everything you put in your body interacts together, and you don't want to find yourself in a toxic overdose situation because of medicine interactions. Your doctor can't guide you if she doesn't know. So put your cards on the table. If she pooh-poohs some of your alternative medicine choices, that's fine. You keep on your path. When your provider starts to see how well you do because you are

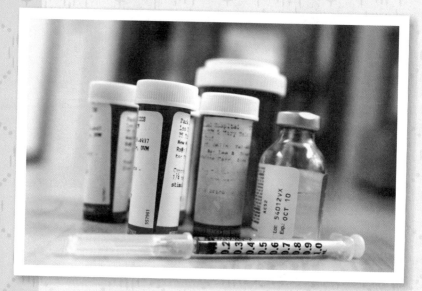

availing yourself of these other treatment modalities, then slowly but surely they will be accepted into mainstream practice. In my lifetime alone, I have seen chiropractic care, osteopathic manipulative medicine, acupuncture, and massage go from being dismissed to being covered by insurance and widely available for inpatients! Medicine is in large part a consumer-driven market. So put it out there with your physicians. The results will speak for themselves.

tip 10:

Inform yourself about your disease. This does not mean you need to go back to school to get a medical degree. It does mean that you should be aware of what's happening in your body. Often, this understanding will help tap into your own inner guidance about steps to take toward healing. The Internet is a wealth of information. But use caution: Facts taken out of context can paint a

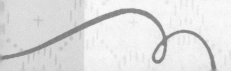

very misleading picture. There is nothing "cookie cutter" or, for that matter, black and white about medicine. How could there be? The human body is a living, breathing thing. I think a more efficient way might be to ask your doctor for some printed material about your diagnosis. If you want more information than that, ask. Because another concern about the Internet is that the source of the information there isn't always clear. It could be distributed by industry (biotech companies, pharmaceutical companies, even insurance companies), and such info is not always unbiased. Your physician will most likely provide you data from the medical literature, which he has evaluated for validity. The Internet is great for getting the basics of your diagnosis under your belt, but for greater detail ask your doc.

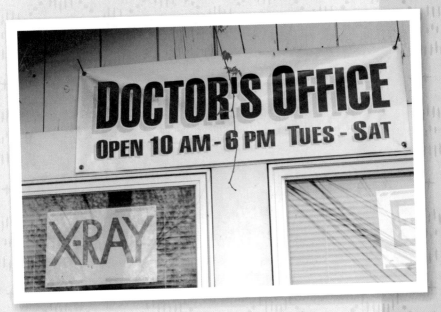

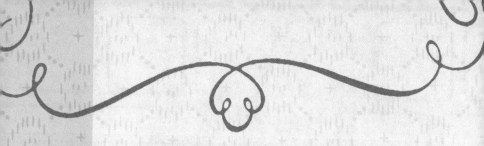

tip 11:

Nurses are your friends. They're hidden gems.
Get the name, number, and e-mail of your physician's nurse. She is your new BFF. Not only is
she a font of information, but she is your inside
track to the Big Cheese, your doctor. She manages,
and manipulates when necessary, the doc's schedule. She can get info to him, with a fairly quick
response. Oncology nurses see it all, and they
know what all the patients are doing for treatment, traditional or otherwise. They are walking
libraries of information. Ask them everything and
anything. I'm willing to bet they will know the
answer. Nurses are huge resources—use them!

tip 12:

Advocate for yourself. This is not to be confused
with being obstinate or obnoxious. It does mean
you should stand up for yourself when the situation warrants it. Doctors do not have all the
answers—a good one will be the first to admit that.
Much of medicine is educated guesswork. But if
in your heart of hearts you just know something
isn't right, push. And then push harder. In the
end, even if we had a perfect health care system,
the only person who can ensure your care is you.
That's a lot of responsibility. Many don't take it. I
encourage you, as overwhelming as it seems, to
take it. It will empower you, free you, yes, even in
some ways heal you, if you do.

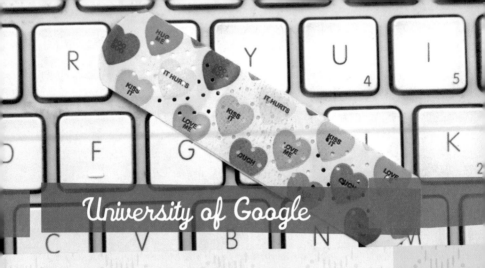

University of Google

Getting organized and setting clear goals will give you peace of mind, help you feel in control, and set you on the path of creating an effective game plan. The Internet is a great place to start learning about your cancer, but it can also be very overwhelming. Move cautiously. Ask a pal to help if you need to. The top ten cancer hospitals are listed online yearly as well as many other useful institutions.

Julie Larson, a young adult services program coordinator with CancerCare (and overall fabulous gal), shares some great advice on how to navigate the Web as well as helpful tips for getting it together CEO style. Hit it, Julie!

TV commercials, news stories, advice from well-meaning friends and family offering their opinion—it all adds up to what people with cancer describe as "too many voices." If you make the decision to dive into the Internet for more information, you may begin wondering, "Can I trust this Web site?" Here is a list of important questions to ask that may help you rely on the information or at least think about it in an informed way.

• What is the purpose of the Web site—educational or commercial? For example, a site sponsored by a pharmaceutical company isn't likely to give you unbiased information about a competing drug. But because that site must meet Food and Drug Administration (FDA) standards, it will be an excellent source on a particular product.

- What is the source of the information? Generally, nationally known cancer centers, medical schools, large nonprofit organizations, and government agencies provide the highest-quality information.
- Are you able to find contact information for the people behind the Web site? If you can't communicate with them, find another source.
- Are the links relevant and appropriate for the site? Sites that refer you to unreliable or frankly commercial sources of information should be rejected.

I always recommend that people focus all their notes, contact, and appointment information in one centralized place. You don't need anything fancy; a simple notebook from the drugstore and a calendar will do the job. Record the name, contact number, date, and a few short notes from important conversations. Begin a calendar for appointments and reminders for when you take medicine.

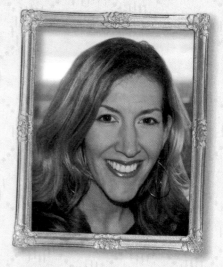

Use a designated folder and notebook for all your medically related information so everything is organized in one place. Write down questions as they come to you, especially the ones that wake

you up in the night. Getting answers to your questions will remove some of the uncertainty and help you feel more in control. Take notes during doctor visits, or ask a family member or good friend to be your secretary during these appointments.

Also, start a log to monitor your side effects through treatment. Everyone tolerates treatment differently. You have to educate yourself on *you* and not get overwhelmed by all the information you read about "possible side effects." Day one is always the first day of a treatment cycle. Record your appetite, energy level, mood, pain, nausea, etc. Do this every day until the next treatment. After a cycle or two of making these notes, most people notice a rhythm to the way their body is tolerating the treatment; this is great information to have. Knowing when you might expect your energy to bounce back or your appetite to return can help you plan for moments when you can do things that help you recharge your batteries. Day one, you may feel great, so you can plan to meet up with friends or spend quality time with your kids. On the other hand, you may find that on day three you tend to be incredibly tired. Knowing this, not scheduling any activities on this particular day of your treatment cycle might be a smart way of taking care of yourself.

Following treatment, ask your doctor for a "Treatment Summary." (Will your doctor know what this is? Probably not. This is a teachable moment when you can explain what you want and why it is important to you as you continue to take control of your health.) This summary should include detailed information about surgeries (and any complications), chemotherapy, radiation (and any significant side effects along with how these effects were managed), and tests that were administered during your treatment phase. This information is important as you move forward after cancer, when health care often becomes more fragmented.

CancerCare

There are so many amazing voices of help and hope in the cancer community. One is CancerCare. These folks are available to anyone—patients, caregivers, and the bereaved—whose life has been impacted by cancer. As they say, the chance to just "talk it through" can sometimes be one of the best ways to understand an overwhelming situation. You can speak with a social worker individually or get connected to a group of others who are facing similar concerns. CancerCare's services support you, give you access to crucial information and help you build personalized strategies for coping—plus they offer financial aid.

How are you doing with ORGANIZATION?

Are you keeping all your reports, medications, insurance information, phone numbers, etc. in one place?

List **five ways** that you will customize your organization and de-clutter your cancer life.

(1)

....

....

....

....

....

....

(2)

....

....

....

....

....

....

....

3

4

5

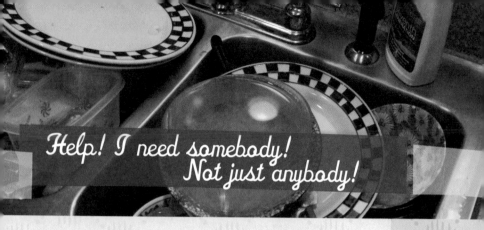

Help! I need somebody!
Not just anybody!

Asking for help can make us feel vulnerable and handicapped. However this is not the time to let your ego stand in the way. This is the time to get resourceful. Don't fall into the trap of not wanting to burden people. You are not an imposition, so ask. Who can lighten your load? The people who love you will be happy to donate their time. More than likely they feel totally helpless and want desperately to contribute. Making your day a little easier is the best gift a person can give and, as we all know, giving is way cooler than receiving. Don't be shy. Organize your needs by making a list and delegating. That's right, coordinate who can do what and when. No task is too big or too small.

If you're unable to call on family or friends, talk with your oncology social worker, network with the nurses, research local organizations with volunteers. Can your church or community of faith assist you? How about that nice neighbor who takes in your FedEx packages when it rains? Get crafty! There are always people who are willing to help, some of whom we barely know or have yet to meet. The trick is to be open to cultivating unexpected relationships and to accept when an offer comes our way.

There are dozens of online organizations that can steer you in the right direction as well. Ah, thank Jesus, Buddha, Elvis, Etc. for Google. For example, the American Cancer Society offers buckets of support including patient navigators. Caring bridge, Care Pages, and Mylifeline.org allow patients to build free personalized Web sites. Your fans (that's right, fans) can view your treatment schedule and life load in order to better help you. They can also post caring messages to lift your spirits when you're down in the dumps.

MySpace and Facebook are also great ways to find cyber pals in a similar situation. I've been surprised by the deeply meaningful relationships I've made by way of the Internet. In some cases, my cyber posse provides more encouragement than the people I have known for decades. Folks who reach out don't think of it as a chore. If the roles were reversed, wouldn't you do the same? So there you go. Enlist your family and friends for support.

What tasks can you *delegate*?
Who can you ask?

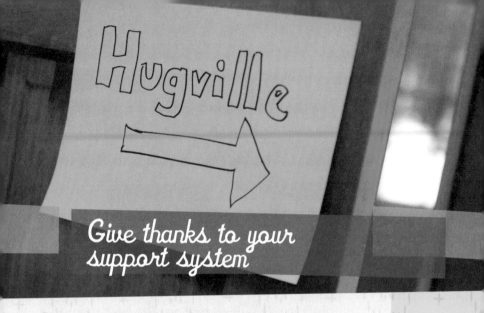

Give thanks to your support system

Just as we think that no one can understand what we go through, the same holds true for the people who hold our hand through the tough stuff. These people are our fierce earth angels and co-survivors. They are the folks who would be your alibi even if you committed the crime. "Did knucklehead do it?" "Nope your Honor." Little does the judge know that your angel drove the getaway car.

When I got sick I moved back in with my parents. I felt thoroughly ashamed about it at the time. All my peers were moving forward while I was running home to Mommy and Daddy. Major buzz kill. And yet I needed to get my head straight and my feet planted. Plus, I was petrified to be alone. My parents lovingly welcomed me in (temporarily). They put their life on hold in the hopes of saving mine. Needless to say I was very lucky.

Often the people closest to us are challenged not only emotionally, but physically, spiritually, and financially. They share your ups as well as your downs. In their private moments, they cry, curse, pray, and tremble. It's very easy to get caught up in our own drama and forget other people's suffering. Though our co-survivors aren't riding the mechanical dragon like we are, standing dangerously close to the flames still leaves them singed. Sometimes we're so busy hanging on for dear life that we can't see how strung out and crispy they've become. Out of nowhere a nasty comment or an exasperated look can start a chain of stress-driven miscommunication.

Your earth angels will have their tantrums and "why mes" too and it's important to let them unload. However don't digest their pain and add more issues to your tissues. Keep it separate. A night off, a weekend away, they too must escape and you must give them permission to do that. We can't succeed in wellness if we're sucking the life out of another.

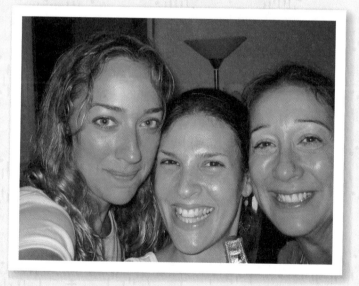

Catch these important people off guard and say thank you. Share how deep your love for them runs. A note, e-mail, lunch or hug will go a long way toward replenishing their energy well. Even if you don't feel like it, make time to put cancer aside and be present for your co-survivors. It will mean more than you know.

Write a thank-you letter
to your co-survivors.

Create a Cancer Posse

Your crew is your healing circle. They are the trusted felines in your pride. In *Crazy Sexy Cancer Tips,* I introduced you to thirteen dynamic babes who rock my world, remind me to laugh, and share their hearts, souls, and secrets. They are the neon swimmies keeping me afloat as I swim in uncharted waters.

Just because you have cancer doesn't mean you don't have regular civilian problems. Add a diagnosis to the mix and *boy* is there plenty to complain about. Your posse knows exactly what you're going through. Still—don't just sit around moaning and shaking. Make healthy commitments with one another to share nutritious dinners, walk or jog in the park, buddy up and join the gym. *Of course* gossip responsibly (remember, karma is a boomerang), be naughty, and swipe the cancer card together, too. Just make sure your posse mission and members support your overall goal of returning to health.

I love witnessing people exchange numbers at my workshops. What a treasure. I feel like Crazy Sexy Big Mama bringin' all the prophets and misfits together. Moments like that remind me of what life is all about—relationships.

Form your own posse as soon as possible, and keep adding to it. Ask your doctor and nurse if they can connect you with other Cancer Babes. Check out other hospitals and support groups in your area or go online and visit me (www .crazysexycancer.com) and other great cancer or wellness communities! We're out there, ya just gotta look. Network with everyone you can think of. Once you start asking and searching, you *will* find other men and women, sometimes right in your own neighborhood. Go out and create your gang, pinkie-swear!

Who's in your posse?

Who do you want in your posse?

Pick up the phone or fire up an e-mail and

START REACHING OUT!

....

....

....

....

....

....

....

....

....

....

....

....

....

....

....

....

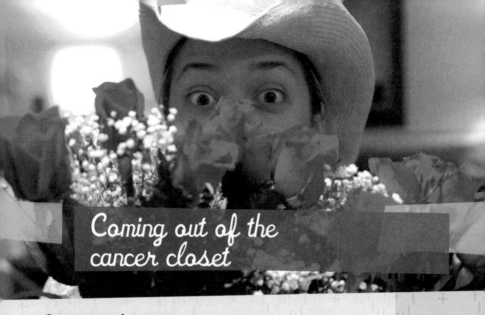

Coming out of the cancer closet

Some cowgirls choose to hide the news, which can be difficult at times, especially when visible signs make your illness more obvious. Others want to write it in the sky. The most important thing to ask yourself is: Will telling this person create more harmony in my life or more dis-ease?

Sharing your cancer tale may lead to an overwhelming feeling of needing to take care of the fragile person in front of you. Once the death-reminder button gets pushed, everyone freaks, not just you. I let a lot of people cry on my shoulder in the beginning, and it was really weird and exhausting.

Take Aunt Lucy (the attention-demanding cat hoarder on your father's side). You pray she never finds out because you know she'll hijack your diagnosis and make it about her. As in all families, there is a scuttlebutt grapevine. Word travels to Aunt Lucy within hours. Overcome with (faux) sorrow she passes out, clonks her head on the coffee table, and gets carried off to the emergency room for stitches. This tap dances on your last nerve and makes you want to do bad things with bad people. Fearing the death threats from your mother, you visit Aunt Lucy and cringe as she proceeds to sob through an entire box of Kleenex (with aloe) tissues. No matter what you say, Aunt Lucy visualizes your hearse idling at the corner. What an energy drain!

In these situations I try to muster the courage to speak up for myself, politely pointing out the inappropriateness of the conversation. You are not responsible for other people's happiness. You can share in their happiness, but you cannot create it. I gave up the happy-maker job long ago, but since I was so good at it my old employers still offer part-time work, especially around the holidays! Stress taxes your immune system. Your job as CEO of you is to do everything in your power to create abundance and health in your life. Anyone who isn't on board gets voted off the island.

What about cancer chats around the office water cooler? That's a tough one, but as you know, a healthy environment at home and at work will greatly contribute to your healing. Sick doesn't necessarily mean ineffective and you may have to demolish that assumption for your obtuse boss. However if your illness is getting in the way of your workflow, then you should have an honest discussion and brainstorm a game plan.

PEOPLE WILL FOLLOW YOUR LEAD. IF YOU DEAL WELL, SO WILL THEY.

If they don't—you are not responsible for mopping up their mania! Be blunt. Nobody knows what to say or how to start the conversation. It's sticky and awkward. But telling your story does get easier over time. Sometimes it helps to come up with a fallback script for breaking the news. Keep a few standard lines and rehearsed answers holstered and ready to fire at a moment's notice.

P.S. Dolling up like a hot tomato helps, too.

script tips

1. Your go-to line is a safety net. Don't feel obligated to dish the specifics. Short and sweet, less is more. Your cancer journey is not a reality TV show where the audience gets to witness your gory details from a safe distance!

2. If you'd rather not talk about it, politely say that today is a cancer-free zone. Puppies, politics, and even prostitution would be delightful topics to discuss. Cancer not so much.

3. Once again, people take their cues from you. If you break the news and melt into a puddle, so will they. I always do my best to talk about my cancer in a bold and confident way. Stick with the facts and ditch the emotion, especially at someone else's party. I do not let cancer unravel me. It is a fact of life (for now). Move on. Pass the crudités. Most people walk away with glazed-over expressions: *Wow, what the hell is wrong with me? If she can cope with cancer then why am I so rattled by my hangnail?* It's a great reality check.

COME UP WITH THREE ANSWERS

to common cancer comments that you can add to
your new script.

....

1 ....

....

....

....

2 ....

....

....

....

....

3 ....

....

....

....

....

faux pas

Folks say the wackiest things. They mean well, they're good people, but sometimes judgment knocks and no one's home. There's a perception that sick looks and sounds a certain way, like if my tumors were on the outside it would make sense. Because they are invisible and I'm sorta pretty, it's awkward. Perhaps I should have a sick person accessory. I could pop an IV pole out of my trunk and wheel it around for clarification.

Here are a few other good ones: "You're too young to have cancer." Brilliant! How about that neurotic calorie-counting office mate who has the gall to tell you that you're lucky? "I've been dieting for years and it's sooo unfair that you get to lose tons of weight effortlessly." Wanna switch? Perhaps your healing plan and choices have been criticized by a friend who continues to plant the "Hey dummy, that won't work" seed. Way to sabotage the sunshine and send me under the covers. I think my next book should be a cancer Miss Manners. Wouldn't that be a gas?

Listen, I know this journey can be downright awful and sad. Don't waste your time enlightening people. Let the assumptions ricochet off your bulletproof vest. Sometimes I wish folks would think before they ask what witty words I'll engrave on my tombstone. Most of the time I just have to laugh—you can, too.

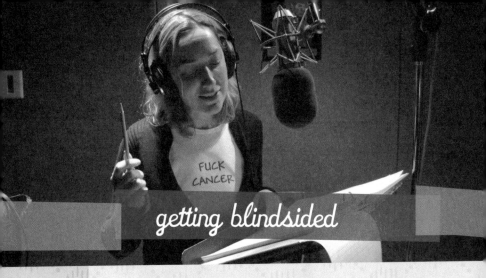

getting blindsided

When I went on my book tour, my publicist gave the local media and radio stations a list of acceptable prep questions. They were ready, and so was I. Most of the interviewers tossed the page into the office shredder, but at least they hovered in the general direction of respectful.

Of course there were a couple of cancer faux pas frontiersmen who opened mouth and inserted foot or cheap high heel. Example: When I showed up for one early show, the host treated me like I had the plague. I fake-sneezed in her direction just to make myself chuckle. Then I asked her to give me the heads-up on what questions she would be asking me. The wench flat-out said no. Huh? Didn't she want the interview to go smoothly? It wasn't like I was asking her to cheat on her SATs.

The crew miked me up, and as the cameras rolled I began to sink in horror as she looked straight down the barrel of the lens with a tragic, car-crash look on her face. "Wow, we're here with Kris Carr, the author and filmmaker who bravely recorded her tragic life and possible death. Good morning, Kris, how are you feeling, dear?" I wanted to stab her in the eye with a shrimp fork, to foam and cuss. I wanted to light her hair on fire with a can of Aqua Net and a Bic lighter. Was she raised in a barn?

DID SHE HAVE A MOTHER WHO TAUGHT HER MANNERS? YOU KNOW, LIKE ELBOWS OFF THE TABLE, SAY PLEASE AND THANK YOU, AND DON'T HARASS THE CANCER CHICK?

I was trapped. Coifed and camera-ready as they zoomed in on my victim close-up. I felt humiliated for catching cancer and for "bravely" sharing my story with the world.

Just then, my sass kicked in. Oh no, not today, Suzie. You are messin' with the wrong babe—and I can play dirty, too. "Wow, that was pretty fucking dramatic for 5 a.m. don't ya think? Good morning, City X, how's it hanging?" Okay, so I didn't say *fucking* OR *how's it hanging* because I was afraid my publishers would tan my hide and they spent a lot of money sending me on the bus-and-truck cancer tour. But damn, I wanted to!

You, too, might get blindsided, but more than likely these incidents will be few and far between. Humor helps tremendously. So do lies! Sometimes when I just don't feel like telling people my story, I pretend that I write about bees. Or that I make porn. That always shuts them up.

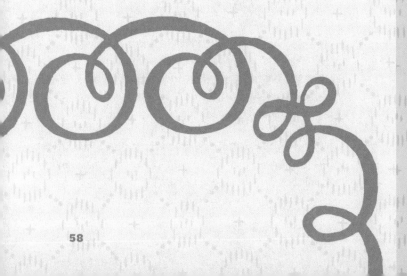

What **CANCER FAUX PAS** have you had thrown at you?
Just for fun, think up a few sassy comebacks that
make you giggle.

....

....

....

....

....

....

....

....

....

....

....

....

....

....

....

....

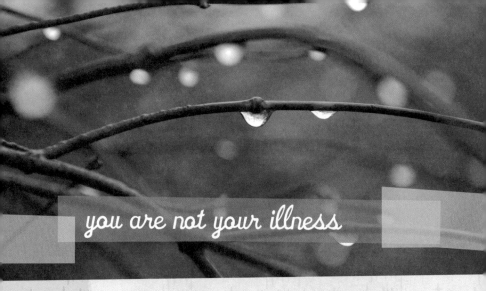

you are not your illness

I hate to admit this, but ever since I let my cancer diagnosis out of the bag I've been bombarded with the standard "Yeah, yeah, you are the bomb but how ya feeling, poor girl?" Even though I have an amazing life with incredible abundance, some people still only see sick. I get those droopy puppy dog eyes and downturned lips from folks who mean well but are just plain annoying. I want to shout, *See beyond the cancer, jackass. I feel fantastic! In fact, last night I hosted an orgy with three steroid-soaked Olympians and a car full of Eastern European strippers, then I ran a marathon, counseled the Dalai Lama, and baked a cake!*

Like it or not sometimes people will see you as your disease. Cancer is still spooky and misunderstood. Recently on my blog, a fine and feisty Cancer Babe giggled while sharing one of her favorite cancer faux pas with me. She had just finished chemo and was swimming laps in a public pool when out of nowhere a crazy mother ran and snatched her child from the water. Apparently my friend's bald head (courtesy of her oncologist) convinced this mother that whatever "that lady" had, her child might catch! Oh, please, are we still stuck in 1950?

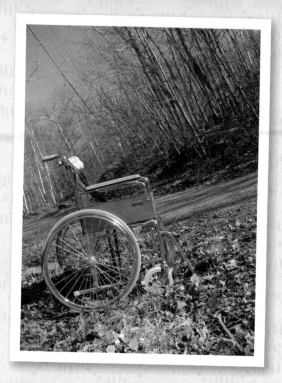

YOU CAN'T CHANGE HOW PEOPLE PERCEIVE YOU, BUT YOU MUST PROTECT HOW YOU SEE YOURSELF.

Don't see sick. See healthy. You are not your circumstances. Your body isn't sick, it's just confused. Look in the mirror; what do you see? No matter what your ego barks out, ask your soul. The ego tends to see fat, flabby, and not "enough." Ego is a little brat! It knows that if you come to your senses, there will be a major coup, and it will no longer rule the roost. Your soul sees radiance and truth.

Take some
fire-engine-red lipstick
(my favorite color is called "I'm Not Really a Waitress")
and write a bunch of positive soul reflections
about yourself on your favorite mirror.
Here are some to get you started:

.... I am GORGEOUS!

.... I am as deep as the ocean.

.... I am a healer.

.... I am a leader.

.... I am a Crazy Sexy
Goddess!

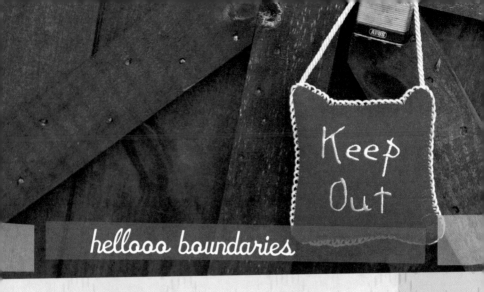

hellooo boundaries

Starting today, things are gonna change. Time for a little housecleaning, and I don't mean with the mop and broom (although a tidy space does create a good healing vibe). I mean your social life. 'Tis the season to trim the fat and put the little black book on a diet. If you're like me, you put other people's needs first and barely address your own. Listen up you Florence Nightingale lunatic, *Cut it out!* The people who really matter will step up to the plate. To the rest: Au revoir, adios, beat it.

LEARN TO SAY THE SEXIEST WORD IN THE UNIVERSE, **NO**.

In fact, let's take a moment and *scream* it right now. *No!* Wow, wow, wow. Say it more darling. The people who drain us like a sink are called vampires. Identify them and get the garlic. Buy a few silver bullets and steal some holy water from the local God house. Protect yourself.

You'll notice that some folks take off when they hear about your big C tragedy (boo hoo). Well, amen. They showed their true colors. Your time is currency; don't bankrupt yourself with selfish victims. This is your life, and I strongly advise you to politely dismiss the naysayers.

I don't mean to diminish how painful this can be. My hope is to turn on a bright light for your clarity. I lost a few very important people in my life as a result of the choices I made post-canSer. Though it cut like a Ginsu at the time, looking back it was a relief. Those wonderful people were never happy with what I gave. They always wanted me to do the friendship their way, the better way. Too much. Kris is Kris. You are you. The cream of the crop will rise to the top. Don't take it personally. This is business, the office of healing to be exact.

Promises Are a Result of Inner "Shoulds"

How often do we overcommit our time? Even though I quack about installing healthy limitations, I'd be lying if I said I always follow my own advice. Sometimes I stink at it, but I'm committed to resisting the "shoulds" because I know my time is precious. Without time, we cannot take care of ourselves and our bliss will always be just around the corner. *As soon as I finish these hundred things I'll have time to be happy.* Nope! When those hundred things are checked off your list, a hundred more will follow. A good model for healthy living was established by the Federal Aviation Administration. That's right, plane rides are loaded with life lessons. Wear your seat belt, don't smoke in the bathroom, and if the plane goes down—put your oxygen mask on *first*.

Challenge your need to please, promise, and give till your fingers bleed. One of my mantras is: Does it tire you or does it inspire you? Ask yourself this very important question and act accordingly. The more you commit to doing things for others, the less time you have for *your* healing adventure. Will you be seen as selfish when you allow other very capable people to take care of themselves? Maybe. But here's the deal: Crumbling under the guilt and cleaning your best friend's garage when you don't feel well isn't taking responsibility for yourself. This is a hard pattern to break because you are an extremely generous person. Perhaps you need to befriend the word *maybe?* While in training, *maybe* is a good word to use. Your next step, we just screamed. What is it? *No!* The step after that is a nasty-dirty, need-some-Ivory-soap-mouth salute. Choose your favorite four-letter zinger, then let loose.

Do an honesty scan and if you really don't want to do something, for God's sake, don't do it! Here's a revolutionary concept: Make *and* keep more promises to yourself. There is a huge difference between self-centered and self-nurturing. Don't confuse them. The plans you make determine how you will spend and fill your life. You are the only one who knows your edge, and you are the only one who can protect it. Without healthy boundaries you will never find balance. Got it?

go ahead—
use the cancer card

Congratulations! You have been preapproved for a Platinum Cancer Card membership! Membership in this ever-growing club does come with its perks, and guess what? No expiration dates. I wish our oncologists offered the same deal! Your Cancer Card is an *I'm human* card, because like it or not you cannot do it all—boundaries, remember? Sometimes just knowing that your card is available in a pinch or on a rainy cancer day can really put your mind at ease.

You may swipe your card freely, but we urge you to use some discretion. Tragically, the card *can* be declined. Therefore, as with all major credit cards, make sure you take the time to read the fine print!

What promises to myself **WILL I KEEP?**
What are some promises I should break?

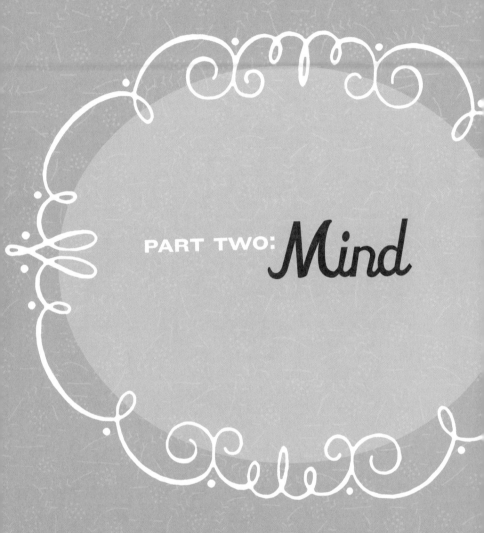

PART TWO: *Mind*

> As the soil, however rich it may be, cannot be productive without cultivation, so the mind without culture can never produce good fruit.
>
> —SENECA

A trained mind is a miraculous mind, so make room for miracles! The old saying, "Don't believe everything you hear" is equally true for the words that rattle around in your head. Welcome to attitude boot camp. As Terri always says: Manifest, visualize, create. Rescue your mind by changing it. This section is about empowering yourself to transform suffering into freedom. The teachings aren't new, however, they have been carefully carved and crafted to suit the needs of glorious CanSer Cowgirls and dudes. So listen up you daring spitfire: Fasten your psychological seat belt and dive, dive, dive. Go deeper than these pages and exercises. Your inner well is bottomless. This is just the beginning, a mere scratch on the surface of your potential. Holy hallelujah!

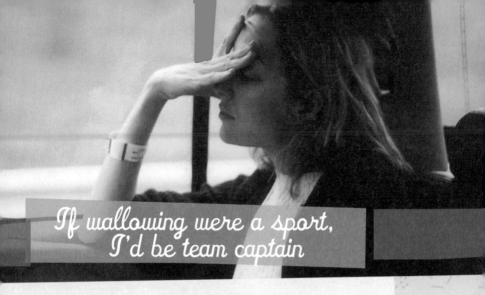

If wallowing were a sport, I'd be team captain

Understanding the complexities of cancer is a full-time job, and none of us applies for the position! You may—no, you will—get the *Why me?* cancer blues, and that's normal and totally expected. Talk it through with someone you trust. Find or hire the strongest shoulder and cry on it. Freak out, wail, spit, and collapse. Yup, pop the pimple and let it ooze. However, be careful not to spiral. Set a limit. Don't give yourself unlimited permission to marinate in misery and become a martyr.

In *Crazy Sexy Cancer Tips* I introduced the Three-Day Rule. Here it is in a walnut shell: Try to explore and indulge the feelings for no more than three days, and then move on. Not to say you can't visit those emotions again. Cancer is a roller coaster: One minute you're up, the next you're plummeting to the ground.

My shrink taught me that cancer patients go through the same post-traumatic stress disorder as soldiers or rape victims. At first I felt guilty about comparing my problems to such a vicious crime. But then I realized she was right, I was in shock and felt completely violated by my own body.

Some medical folks may tell you that you might become deeply depressed or anxious during or after treatment. Others have no concept of what truly goes on in the mind of a survivor. Even though they see the effects of cancer every day they still don't get it. Oncologists are still human, they can get caught up in stigmas too. Many of them still don't recognize that the cancer has become more chronic and manageable.

TODAY MORE PEOPLE ARE LIVING WITH DISEASE. AND THESE SURVIVORS NEED TO BE TREATED AND COUNSELED DIFFERENTLY. WELLNESS ISN'T BLACK-AND-WHITE.

Regardless of whether you've made it through the mine field or are still dodging bullets, welcome back from your own personal Vietnam. Like many of those brave soldiers, you may feel that there is no place for you. It could be that family and friends imagine that you are exaggerating the toll your "battle" has taken on you. Well, guess what? They're wrong. When you've been to the border of your mortality, a little loving rehabilitation is damn well in order!

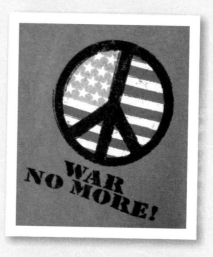

How do you find stability in the midst of unsafety?

THE VERY FIRST THING THAT COMES TO YOUR MIND IS A GUT MESSAGE.

Incorporate it into your life on a regular basis.

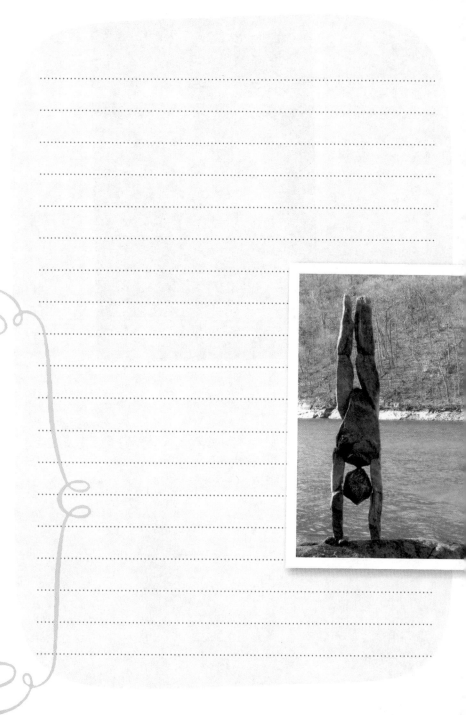

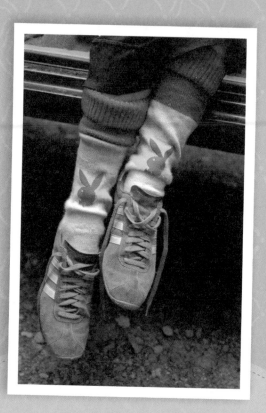

I feel naked and abandoned. I do my very best. I work so hard to "let go" of all the nasties in me, to do the "right" thing, and yet here I am drifting in a shit storm! I'd crawl on broken glass to go back, but I know I can't. So what should I do? How do I tie my shoe so that I can take one step forward?

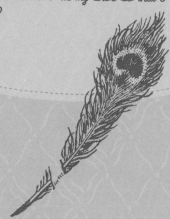

checkup from the neck up

Some of your feelings may seem totally irrational, but underneath the ridiculous there always lies an important nugget. Therapists, support groups, and Cancer Posses can help. I went through a phase in which so-called healthy people made me bitter. I judged everybody: Look at the jackass at twelve o'clock. *He's* chain smoking and *I'm* the one with cancer? Or how about the carcinogenic hot dog–eating bimbo at work? How come *she* doesn't have to find the humor in the tumor just to get by? The worst is when you see a person that's just pure child-molesting, granny-hunting bad. That's the biggest slap in the face. It can be really depressing to be the "sick" chick. While everyone else builds castles in the sandbox, you're banished to the outside holding your pink plastic shovel and a pail full of cancer cooties.

Here's what Crazy Sexy posse babe Terri has to say about the slippery slope called depression.

There are many reasons cancer survivors may be vulnerable to depression. When I was diagnosed, I was sad and angry that my innocence—the *it will never happen to me* phase of my life—was abruptly cut short. I struggled with integrating my diagnosis with my self-image of being strong, able to handle anything, and *healthy*. This took time and work with a fantastic therapist. I looked at therapy as a gift I could give myself. One hour a week with a person who did not need me to be anyone or anything for her . . . an hour to acknowledge my fear without the fear that she would fall apart. (Of course I *am* a therapist, so I did not have the resistance to seeking help that many others may have.)

So let's talk ways to manage depression. A huge pitfall to be aware of is the danger of over-exaggerating. We all do it—it's a current popular speech trend in this country. But there is a danger in not talking straight. How many times have you uttered the phrases, "I just can't take another second of . . . having the worst day ever . . . nothing ever goes right in my life . . ." Realistically, none of these statements is true at any given time. And none of these statements—or the pessimistic thinking at their base—is something you want to reinforce in your life.

I had a personal experience with the challenge of not overexaggerating when I got into family therapy with my husband and our three boys. They had lost their mom years before, and I had married the whole kit and kaboodle of angry, acting-out teens. The therapist noted in session one that we were a family that did not talk "straight" . . . huh? I was confused until she pointed out how sarcastic and exaggeratedly all of us spoke. She explained

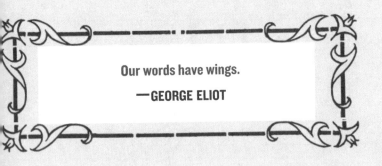

Our words have wings.
—GEORGE ELIOT

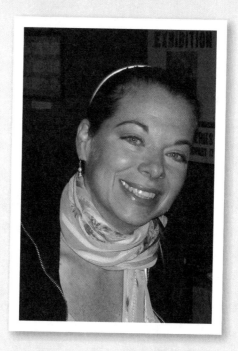

that it was a way to veil the hostility we were feeling. The positive changes that happened within my family system from just learning to "talk straight" were amazing.

The power of realistic vocabulary to help fight depression is great. What will *really* happen if you don't meet that deadline or make it to that meeting? As cancer survivors, we are truly dealing with life and death; missing any meeting or deadline will surely not end your life. I have a *then what* exercise I do with my clients. It is an invitation to play out the catastrophic fantasy until it loses power over you. To be aware of negative overexaggerating is to be more authentic in your language and in your life. This alleviates mental stress and gives you more brain space for the good stuff.

Here are some more tips to help you out:

tip 1:

Essential oils do your brain good. There are many amazing essential oils out there that do an array of things. I use them with my clients as a mood lifter. Lavender—my favorite—is amazing for lessening anxiety, depression, and insomnia. Use it anytime you need a lift in mood. Take five deep breaths of the oil while visualizing breathing in positive peaceful energy and exhaling negativity, stress, and depression. Buy a meditation CD (I like Dr. Brian Weiss's tapes on meditation, relaxation, and regression) and commit twenty minutes a day to listening to that CD and breathing in your oil. Over time you will train your body to associate complete relaxation and good feelings with your essential oil; when you are out and about in the stressful world, one whiff and your body will respond by relaxing and releasing stress.

tip 2:

Move your booty. Or as Kris says in *Crazy Sexy Cancer Tips*, shake your ass! Exercise is another extremely effective tool in the fight against depression. Do not set yourself up to fail. You don't have to participate in an Ironman. You just have to move. Commit to twenty minutes a day of walking briskly. Get a pal to go with you (it is harder to blow it off with your friend waiting for you on the corner of 82nd and Broadway)—it will lift your mood and increase the serotonin levels in your brain.

tip 3:

Do your morning pages. Write write write and then . . . write some more. Julia Cameron talks about the healing effect of writing "morning pages" in her book *The Artist's Way*. She suggests that you wake up and write three unedited pages before your green tea, before your superego has a chance to change what you would write . . . before the "shoulds" wake up. It is a morning mind dump that will clear your head of clutter and negativity. Honor yourself with some sacred a.m. time; you'll feel lighter and better for it.

tip 4:

You are not a bear . . . so don't hibernate. Social interaction with supportive friends and family is a must . . . even when you don't feel like it. Being with people who love you feeds the soul. Ask for what you need from the close relationships in your life. Maybe it's just a back massage or an empathic ear to listen and *not* fix anything. Be clear and honest about what you can and cannot do. Don't be committed to the false self for everyone else's sake. This is exhausting and alienating to you. Tell the truth . . . it really will help.

tip 5:

Most important . . . never give up hope. Know that your effort to feel better will pay off. Take these tools, use them, and come up with your own winning formula. Know that you are the only person on this planet with your DNA. There will only ever be one you. You matter; you're worth the effort to work for a happy and fulfilled life. Just decide you won't take no for an answer *no matter what!*

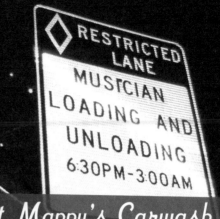

RESTRICTED LANE
MUSICIAN LOADING AND UNLOADING
6:30PM–3:00AM

story time at Manny's Carwash

One of my favorite jobs in New York City was as a cocktail waitress at a legendary blues bar named Manny's Carwash. I learned more about the life of an artist from the world-class musicians in that smoky dive than I ever did studying acting or painting in college. (I also learned a lot about Quaaludes, but that's another story.) The blues lit me up. They made me imagine sultry summer nights on the bayou. Broken promises, bad cases of love, sneaking around, stormy Mondays, and naked angels were the standard—in the key of G. The life of a blues musician—especially a sideman—is tough. It's full of booze and ramen noodles. Most of the legends I met played as a salve. If they didn't strum that 1,3,5 chord progression, their heart would break and they'd die.

One particular wrinkly old man made a deep impression on me. I can't remember his name, but I can still see his weathered face. Let's call him Old Ronny Holmes for the sake of the story. Ronny must have been in his late seventies, early eighties, and man could that cat howl and blow a harmonica. He was one of the last of a generation of unknown greats, dignified hustlers who always wore three-piece suits but couldn't pay their bar tabs.

Ronny would stop by my station and charm me into pouring top-shelf Courvoisier XO (extra old) in exchange for a good story. "Krissy"—for some reason all the blues dudes called me Krissy—"did I ever tell you the story of my grandpappy's goat?"

"No, Ronny, you didn't, but I'd sure like to hear it," I'd reply.

He'd rub his hands together and tell me to pour him a *tall* glass, no being stingy. "Back in Mississippi on my pappy's farm," he'd begin, "there lay a deep hole behind the barn. Pappy was fixin' to put in a new well come spring, but for years the seasons came and went with no sign of a well.

"One day us grandkids noticed that pappy's favorite goat had gone missin'. Well, we practically tore the place apart looking for the damn thing, until we just gave out. 'Must of been snatched up by a coyote,' Pappy said. Little did we know that the damn goat had fallen into the deep hole. At the same time, after listening to all my granny's complaints about the dangers of small children tearing 'round near the hole, my pappy reluctantly agreed to fill it.

"The next day old man Spencer came over with his John Deere backhoe and proceeded to dump mounds of dirt down the hole and onto the head of Pappy's goat. When the dirt landed, Pappy's goat would shake it off and stamp it down. The more dirt that fell on that creature, the more he would shake it off and stamp it down until finally he shook it off, stamped it down, and rose right out of that hole."

Ronny was a wise old man, and so was his grandpa's goat. To this day I believe he knew that I needed to hear that story. For years I have been shaking it off and stamping it down. Now it's time to rise.

Mood Lube

Our mental state really changes our physical condition, but sometimes we all need a helping hand to get back in the saddle. This isn't about the sprint—it's about the long haul. Yoga, exercise, healthy food, nature and therapy will all help. However, when we're still struggling, some mood lube (aka medication) can be a good tool to push us over the hump. If you're in crisis, it's important that your pain get managed. There is nothing wrong with a little pharmaceutical relief, especially if you're doing soul work to go with it. I spent years of my life stoking the fires of depression and anxiety. I'd suffer the side effects of a girl spinning out of control. With medical guidance I decided to take Prozac. Those pills were like a sturdy pair of boots protecting my ankles from the rocky ground. Every day we decide how to use our time and energy. Use it wisely. Give yourself permission to accept help when you feel helpless. Your inner mother is wise so listen to her.

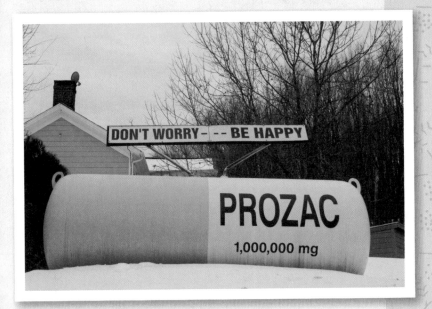

What is your *inner mother* telling you?

WKDC Radio
[my initials—you insert yours]

Your brain is a radio transmitter. It broadcasts thoughts, directions, and vibrations to your cells, and you get to choose the station it's tuned to. Is your DJ a Hell's Angel or a minister? Are you playing soulful classics or blaring death metal? Even worse, are you rocking back and forth to the sound of white-noise static?

Thoughts are electrical currents that send messages to your body. Deepak Chopra, renowned physician, best-selling author, spiritual leader, and very snazzy dresser, says, "If you have happy thoughts, then you make happy molecules." Deepak's studies of mind–body medicine indicate that there is a healing power beyond what Western science can explain. He calls this energy quantum healing: "Our bodies ultimately are fields of information, intelligence, and energy. Quantum healing involves a shift in the fields of energy information, so as to bring about a correction in an idea that has gone wrong."

How do you feel when you're jealous or, worse, envious? Wildly enraged? Deeply insecure? Unfortunately, stinking thinking spoils the party and makes you a downer. No one wants to hang out or be around you—and the person who suffers the most is you.

Now think about the light. How do you feel when you are beaming with pure shazizzle? When there is no doubt in your mind that you will be president, heal the planet, cool global warming, and receive a billion-dollar check from those generous saints at Publishers Clearing House? You feel *awesome!* Both of these states affect your mind and your body. Both are something you choose. Now, I'm not saying you have to be bliss-boy or -babe 24/7.

SOMETIMES MAD-SAD-RAGE IS THE TICKET TO SELF-PRESERVATION AND LIBERATION.

But take note and then send positive energy to the source of the pain. Remember, you are what you eat, drink, and think.

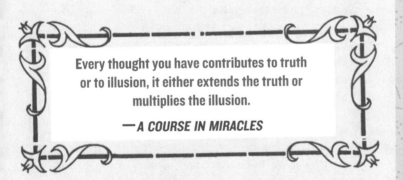

Every thought you have contributes to truth or to illusion, it either extends the truth or multiplies the illusion.

—*A COURSE IN MIRACLES*

What station is your brain tuned to?
What's on your playlist?
Who are your DJs?

Good Vibrations

Dr. Ginger Southall was one of my favorite teachers at the Hippocrates Health Institute, the amazing healing center where I received my Holistic Health Educator certification. Check out how she takes the inner radio station to a whole new level in excerpts from an article she wrote titled "Quantum Leaps in Healing," first published in *Hippocrates: Saving Our World* magazine.

Take it away, lovely Dr. Ginger . . .

Our brains are not just organs encased in our skulls, but rather the most powerfully complex electrical energy instruments ever known to man. Through the stimulation of various brain centers our organs, glands, heart, voluntary, and involuntary movements are all controlled. That's a concept we all can understand. What most people are not familiar with is the connection between our body's "thought vibrations" and the rest of our life, including our health.

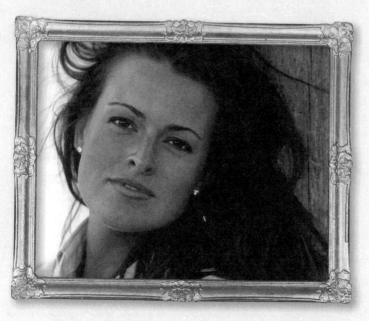

Every thought you have has a frequency or vibration. Your thoughts actually send out magnetic energy. You've probably experienced "thought energy" a thousand times in your life but didn't even know it. Think about it. How many times have you been around someone who is unpleasant and you just don't want to be in their presence? You may get "bad vibes" about that person because of their pessimism and "negative energy." But then there's that person you love to be around; they are always upbeat, positive, and have a zest for life. Their optimism and "good vibes" make you feel good.

Even the former head of the FDA's Office of Drug Evaluation, Robert DeLap, MD, concedes, "Expectation is a powerful thing . . . the more you believe you're going to benefit from a treatment, the more likely it is that you will experience a benefit."

So how can you put this information into action; ignite success in all areas of your life, especially your health? Wrap your mind around the idea that whatever path you choose to take on your road to wellness should at the very least involve you working with your own mind, your thoughts, and your emotions. Live a life full of good intentions, gratitude, faith, forgiveness, and joy and you will watch miracles become a daily happening in your life.

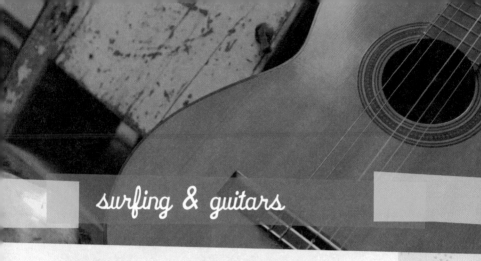

surfing & guitars

Make a list of ten activities or dreams that make you wiggle and send jolts of electricity up your spine. Make sure they are doable. "I want to be a pro surfer today" is a reach. "I want to learn how to surf"—hooray! Here's a board, start paddling! Write down the first things that come to mind and post it someplace where you can see it. Don't get stuck in practicalities, and don't edit. Your only limitation is your imagination. Maybe you've always wanted to play the guitar. Can you pick one up at the flea market? If the answer is yes, then take it to the next level and answer that ad in the paper—you know, the one from the cute (yet way too young for you, Mrs. Robinson) music teacher who lives five minutes from your house.

I love cooking, and I instinctively knew that my kitchen would become my pharmacy once cancer invited itself to dinner. At first I borrowed the money from my folks to take some classes and learn the basics. Pretty soon I was back in school studying nutrition, and now I love teaching others all that I've learned. For some people, reading a good book is like a Calgon bubble bath—it takes you away. Perhaps there's a swanky book club you can join. Better yet, start one of your own. Trailblazers take initiative. So be a leader and enlist your friends to join you. Create a syllabus drenched with romping sex and protest. How fun your weekly assignment will be!

I've found that the best way to overcome fear is to actively change my focus—to redirect my energy so that it flows in a positive direction. As I mentioned in the introduction, creativity has always been my bounding river. So I became a filmmaker instead of a patient, an author instead of a victim. You don't have to be good at what you choose. In fact, go ahead and embrace being rotten. You already have cancer; why would bongos intimidate you?

SO WHAT'S YOUR PASSION? WHAT TURNS YOU ON? WHATEVER IT IS, CHANNEL SOME LOVE AND FIRE IN THAT DIRECTION.

If you're thinking that this is an ass-backward place to start, you're wrong. It's all part of the master plan for liberation. Pivot your attention and find your bliss. Just because you have cancer doesn't mean you can't enjoy life. Haven't you already warehoused yourself enough? Reality check: If you keep blowing off your life, your life will thank you with an equal invitation.

I promise cancer won't always be your first and last thought of the day. As life returns to normal, you may come to accept that, like it or not, cancer is just another thing you have to roll with. It might even become an interesting piece of the puzzle that makes you utterly fabulous and fascinating!

> Follow your bliss. The heroic path is living the individual adventure. Nothing is exciting if you know what the outcome will be. To refuse the call means stagnation.
>
> **—JOSEPH CAMPBELL**

Go ahead, start your list.
Ten things you want to try.

Whatever blows your skirt up—write it.
Then do it. Oprah and Madonna don't let their
wishes sit in a book, so why should you?

1

2

3

4

5

6

7

8

9

10

11

12

13

be a crayon-wielding van gogh

How many decades have passed since you allowed yourself the therapeutic joy of doodling? Art isn't just for skinny people in berets and black turtlenecks. Art is healing. Place a pack of colored pencils and a sheet of paper in front of any child and voilà. Do the same thing with grown-ups and you'll witness an endless display of insecurities and resistance. Grown-ups are very serious people. They are domesticated to wipe out the whimsy. The piano is boarded up, that chapter of life is over. But you are an artist, a highly imaginative creative spirit. Your very existence is an expression of beauty. Forget about quality and instead savor the pleasure of the process. Get this: Studies show that creativity can drastically reduce stress levels and pain perception. In fact, art, prayer, and healing are associated with similar brain wave patterns. How cool!

Creativity allows you to take a break from that which ails you. It also serves as a way to process your experience. Art gets the pain out of your body and gives it shape and words. It mends the broken heart that aches over cancer. Honor your need to express yourself. This doesn't mean you have to try to follow Bob Ross patiently stroking out a mountain in reruns of *The Joy of Painting* on PBS. Think of art as an important tool in your healing process and allow yourself some playtime with your muse.

What did you love to do when you were a kid?
Did you find magic in cutting out paper snowflakes and taping them to the fridge? I did.

LIST THREE WAYS TO INSPIRE YOUR INNER VAN GOGH.

1 ....
....
....

2 ....
....
....

3 ....
....
....
....

It took me four years to paint like Raphael,
but a lifetime to paint like a child.

—PABLO PICASSO

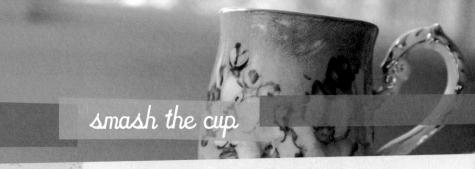

smash the cup

Yes, it blows that you have cancer, but is everything in your life diseased? I don't think so, hot stuff. Just say no to emotional metastasis! That's right: Don't let cancer poison your entire world. It's easy for all the good stuff to get buried under the weight of chemo, radiation, surgery, dirty toilets, and stuffed gutters. But we choose our focus. Is your cup half full or better yet brimming over? Do you complain about its size and shape on a daily basis? Smash your perception of the leaky, half-empty cup. Do it right now. Let this exercise be an outlet to release some bottled up tension. Grab a pretty cup, one you really love, and smash it on your kitchen floor! Huh? Why smash a good cup; why not direct your aggression towards a chipped one that reads #1 golfer? Because when the universe asks us to let go of our attachments and grow, discomfort is sure to arise. Our half-empty cups are protective mechanisms employed by our ego's desire to keep us in line: "Life sucks. Stick with me and we'll bitch together."

We all love excuses. We love to dodge responsibility, complain, and pout. We constantly blame the world cheating us. Is it weird to think that sometimes we adore our desperation? Why stay in a destructive relationship or devour a bag of sugar if we know that these decisions will only make us sad? Many of us find comfort in the chaos because at least it's predictable.

Clearly, what we've been trained to love doesn't always serve our best interests. Wake up! You no longer need to cling to your negative thoughts like a high school sweetheart. There is no protection in that space. Drama-love is a convenient excuse for remaining stuck. Time to break up and move on. So smash that nice half-empty cup already!

"The Secret," CanSer Cowgirl Style

"Without exception, every human being has the ability to transform any weakness or suffering into strength, power, perfect peace, health, and abundance." Exactly! What a lovely reminder brought to us by the mega hit *The Secret*. Perhaps you've watched this film, read the book, or heard similar tapes on the subject. But did you listen?

Negative thoughts create negative energy and negative realities. Positive thoughts and energy bring happiness and abundance into our lives. Happiness is heaven, and heaven is here on earth. You've heard this simple concept many times I'm sure. You may even be rolling your eyes and reaching for the barf bucket. Yet you know it's true. So what holds you back from strengthening your manifestation muscle on a daily basis? See your dreams. Hear them, taste them, become them. I know from my own experience that when my focus is weak I lose track of my needs. I overwork, underplay, and allow other people's agendas to overtake mine. Once I'm adrift it's very easy to be devoured by doubt stoking the fires of failure and all the fears that accompany it. To get unstuck from this cemented place we must do one simple yet profound action: Change our minds.

Have you ever set a really clear intention? Not a "hope"—hopes are too wishy-washy roulette for my taste. Roll the dice and "hope" you win. Hmmm, success seems pretty random under this model. Instead, stack the odds in your favor with directed and nurtured thought. Intentions place your desires on a course for success. We don't just toss our desires out to the "universe" and then forget. We lovingly raise them like little children.

To successfully manifest your dreams you must be able to feel the emotion that accompanies the desire. If you want to be healthy, then imagine how healthy feels. Really put yourself there. What else do you need to make your life better? More money for organic veggies, the perfect job with benefits, a relationship with a hot yet spiritually advanced partner? Soak yourself in the physical sensations of abundance. Get specific and detailed.

What you hold in your mind you can create. But here's the catch: You must back up your wants and desires with a willingness to meet the universe halfway. Sitting on your ass and dreaming won't get you to the finish line. Get busy! Brainstorm like you've never brainstormed before. What concrete steps can you take regardless of your condition? Big or small, doesn't matter. What matters is that you move the energy towards your desired outcome. Success is six degrees of separation. I guarantee you know someone or something that can help you network. But keep your purdy peepers open! Sometimes you will receive what you intend in a different package. Though it may look like the polar opposite of what you thought it would be, accept the gift anyway. You will not be sorry.

A gorgeous way to support our intention and reinforce these important teachings is by constantly filling our lives with uplifting and spiritually informative reading material, CDs, DVDs, etc. Surround yourself with the sacred. Don't wait for the guru to come to you. An inspirational electric community fills in the gaps between visits to the yoga studio, mosque, or wizard college. Each time we study spiritual texts, we get another diamond. Wear them. Gems can't shine in a box. Create a syllabus and school yourself. Try to refrain from being a one-note simpleton, "Jesus or else!" The original hippie wouldn't like that very much. We expand our God knowledge to include different philosophies and traditions not to replace our spiritual beliefs, but to deepen them. Sadly in many cases religion has lost its spirituality. Like a big cosmic pizza pie, we've carved up slivers of God and claimed that our piece is the tastiest. Dogma and doctrine break the divine connection. When God is only "out there" we will always feel powerless and small.

In times of crisis I haul ass to my teachers. However, as my plucky therapist says, crisis isn't the only time we can grow. Why wait till we are at the bottom and the only place to go is up?

What if we worked on our "how to be a happy human" studies on a consistent basis? Here's what would happen: At the end of every year of your life you would be a truly better person. That's right, at your yearly bliss evaluation you would pat yourself on the back and say, "Go girrrrl, look at me, one step closer."

I myself have a long way to go—a (long) lifetime to be exact—and that's wildly exciting. The most inspiring aspect of reminders like "The Secret" isn't what they say, it's the sheer number of people saying the exact same thing from their own unique perspective. Countless faiths and sciences come together through cinema with the intention of reflecting the collective consciousness back to us. Bravo!

A few favorite *Secret* diamonds:

- **You will attract according to your belief.**

- **Visualize and materialize. Our job is not to figure out how. The how will show up out of a commitment and belief in the what.**

- **Disease can't live in a healthy body, so see yourself living in a healthy body.**

- *Incurable* **means "curable from the inside."**

- **You are the author of your destiny. The pen is in your hand.**

Watch the flick yourself, or read the book. Then crack open your journal and jot down the quotes that inspired you. Soak in the meaning behind those quotes and begin to locate tangible ways to incorporate their messages into your life. When you're done, pick another flick and turn another page. Dig deeper. Just one other thing (because the title of this section is "The Secret CanSer Cowgirl Style"): it's important to remember that though we often attract our successes and our failures, we didn't attract cancer. The objective of these teachings and of all the advice in this book is simple. Retrain your brain.

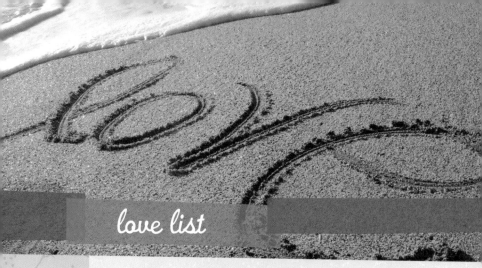

love list

Love is a magnetic force that attracts an infinite amount of goodness into our cells. Love makes us radiant and tipsy with joy. In times of stress or trauma, however, it can be hard to locate the love. Identify what you love. Give your darlings props no matter how small or seemingly insignificant. This simple act reminds us that life is too sweet to be bitter. Make a list and watch it grow. Love is innocent, it thrives off of acknowledgment just like we do. It's amazing how many beautiful things we notice when we take the time to look.

Notice the love and invite it to tea. Don't be a one-dimensional cancer patient. Monotonous city! If you play the cancer, cancer, cancer tape, then that's all you'll get back. When I was an actress in New York, I did my best to avoid the out-of-work actors (such as myself). Most of us were so desperate and blinded by our blood-thirst for fame that we saw nothing of the world around us: War. *Huh?* Darfur. *Is that a new theater?* Global warming. *I know, I hate that, too. Makes me sweat my makeup off.* Cancer. *Eww, total crimp in my style. Can I bum a cigarette?* Among my fellow thespians, I knew who would rise to stardom by how broad their focus was. If they read the paper, had a hobby, and talked about more than themselves, chances were they'd get work. The me, me, me, the-world-revolves-around-me types were shoo-ins for the unemployment line.

I love writing the word "love" in the sand

Catching fireflies and then letting them go

Colored Sharpies

My kitty

Scrabble (even though I am bad at it)

Post-it notes

Saying I went to Harvard when I didn't

Gossiping with my sister

Claw-foot tubs

A boot filled with posies

Chet Baker and kalamata olives

Watching Discovery Channel with my dad

Sweatpants

Rhinestone hair clips

Mechanical pencils

Jazzercise

Doodling in the columns of official documents

Dancing with my friend Vera

Access Hollywood

Taking ten matchbooks on my way out of a restaurant

The New Yorker

When my husband cleans the juicer

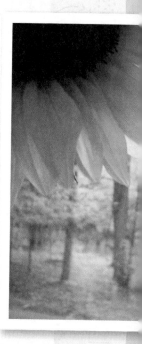

What soul-fortifying things do you love?
WRITE YOUR LOVE LIST HERE:

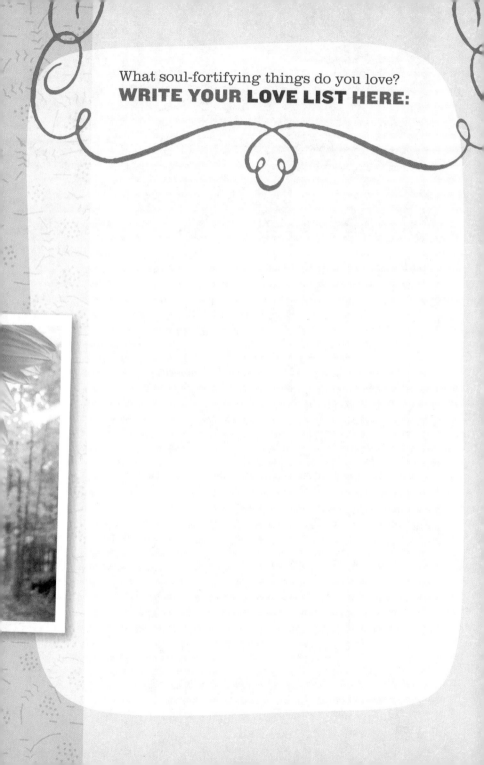

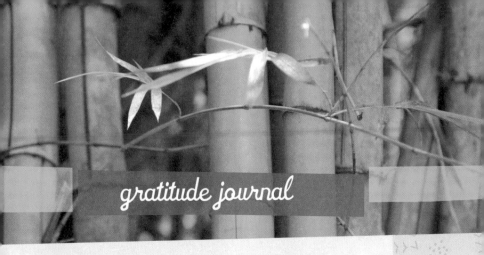

gratitude journal

Now that you've identified what you love, it's a delicious time to welcome a relationship with gratitude into your life. Have you ever noticed that when you choose to be thankful you receive more to be thankful for? Gratitude puts us in a position of having instead of wanting. When I take stock of my blessings, I get more blessings. When I throw bottomless "wanting" out into the universe, the only thing I get back is more wanting. The universe is so kind! Just as with our love list and the power of intention, notice what you do have instead of focusing on what you don't. Plenty multiplies like horny bunnies, but so does lack. What bunny do you choose?

Look around you. A child's laughter or your best friend's funny phone messages, the hot water you used for your shower and the good parking space at Target. The list is endless. Open your eyes. If you see nothing then you've been hijacked by your inner sourpuss. This is very serious. Immediately send a SWAT team armed with a fire hose of sunshine to your rescue.

A great way to start this dialogue is with a gratitude journal. My journals are the match to the tinder of my creativity. I chat, pray, and set clear intensions for the universe to work on. As we've discussed, the universe loves that. Less stuff for it to figure out!

A written prayer of thanks works like a charm. Instead of *"Please make it go away now!"* I say, "Thank you for my perfect health, wealth, and happiness." My life is abundant *now;* rivers of joy and health flood my inner ashram and fill me with stamina, strength, and amen. Life doesn't start at the end of the cancer rainbow, it's happening right now. So don't waste it, love. Holy growth rodeo! Can you imagine how empowered you could feel if nothing held you back? Acknowledge the scratchy stuff, but don't let it tear your skin off. That simple shift in perception can transform your life.

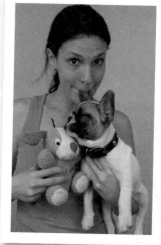

Leslie and handsome Pierre

Think about this: What if the cancer disappeared today? Would you be instantly happy? Tell the truth. My sense is that the answer would be no. Most of us build state-of-the-art infrastructure to house our misery. We provide sturdy platforms for doubt, depression, and despair. If the main source of the misery were removed, don't think for a nanosecond that the self-created support beams would vanish with it.

For me, it's too overwhelming to focus on the source of my ouchies all the time. Instead I focus on creating a different type of inner support system: changing my diet, being kind to myself, exercising, writing in my gratitude journal, bathing myself with affirmations, getting a massage, creating doable lists and establishing protective boundaries, plus all the other gems in this book.

When you stop feeding and supporting cancer, it can, and sometimes will, collapse. You may wake up one morning and realize that it has been minutes, hours, days, weeks, months, or even years since you thought about it. Brava! You are in control again. You're doing your work, and the transformation is so bright that we all need Prada sunglasses. Good for you!

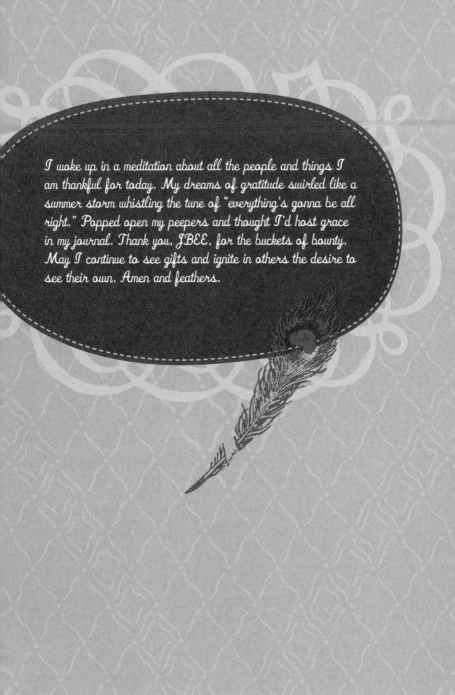

I woke up in a meditation about all the people and things I am thankful for today. My dreams of gratitude swirled like a summer storm whistling the tune of "everything's gonna be all right." Popped open my peepers and thought I'd host grace in my journal. Thank you, JBEE, for the buckets of bounty. May I continue to see gifts and ignite in others the desire to see their own. Amen and feathers.

Traffic Violations

After you read this section, grab your coat and speed (at least 75 miles per hour) to your favorite stationery store. If you don't have one, find one. If you can't leave the house, go online. If you can't go online, staple a stack of napkins together. Your mission is to find (or make) the most delicious journal that will inspire you to split open and let it rip! This journal is a no-lies-fly zone. Only reality, truth, and positive words are contained within its pages. You can use this for two purposes only: gratitude and affirmations. You cannot fill these pages with lists, complaints, daily summaries, or spinning wheels. Got it? *Note:* A groovy pen really helps.

NOW FIND A COMFORTABLE CHAIR, TURN DOWN THE NOISE, AND QUIET YOUR INSIDES.

Light a candle and exhale. Begin to write down a list of things you are grateful for in the present tense, even if they haven't materialized yet. Feel the love and comfort of already having what you desire. Say thank you for

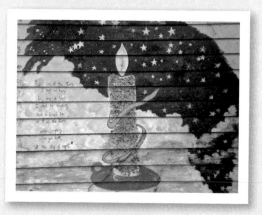

answered prayers as if they have happened. Broadcast healing thoughts and requests to the universe. So often we curse the seeds that didn't take hold, yet we fail to realize that it wasn't their season. Two years later you look in the garden and voilà, a red rose. My friend (and righteous babe) Marianne Williamson ends many of her spiritual talks and prayers with the powerful words *and so it is*. Captain Picard from *Star Trek* employed a similar tactic when he thundered, "Make it so, Number One." Make it so.

If and when you spiral into helplessness, grab your gratitude journal and redirect your attention. Take inventory of your wealth instead of validating your poverty. How great do you feel when a person genuinely appreciates the work you've done for her? What about when you bust your hump and that wench didn't even notice? Focus on the work you've done for yourself, the work the universe is doing for you right now, and leave room for the magic you don't even know about.

This exercise will give you an attitude makeover. Commit to doing it regularly. If you do, your life will change. You will not be the same person. Saying thanks will strap you to JBEE's (Jesus, Buddha, Elvis, Etc.) jumper cables and charge your battery.

I am so grateful that we humans woke up and came to our senses in protection of Mama Earth and all her wee ones. We realized that there is no separation and that our part equals the big-picture whole.

I am grateful that we retracted our knives and instead chose to extend hands of peace to hold our brothers and sisters around the world and especially in the Middle East.

I am grateful that money is silly and that real currency is exchanged with a smile.

I am grateful for parents who taught me I could do anything and a mom who believes in the transformative power of sock monkeys.

I am grateful for a husband who is my best friend.

I am grateful for in-laws who hold grandparent wisdom and notice the birds.

I am grateful that a feather on the ground is a sign that the universe just answered a prayer.

I am grateful for the opportunity to serve.

I am grateful for fantastic bowel movements!

I am grateful for my friends and for the people I don't like so much because they remind me to release my attachment to simple thinking.

I am grateful for my kitty.

I am grateful for all the blessings in my life, and I am proud of myself for actually seeing and acknowledging them.

I am grateful for each of you, all the CanSer Cowgirls and dudes who are seekers of truth, health, and real-deal happiness.

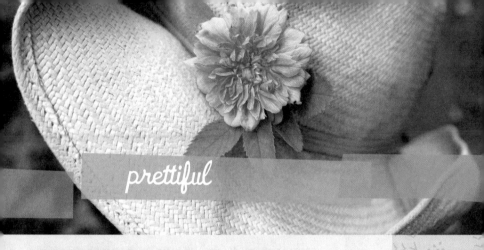

prettiful

REMEMBER WHEN WE WERE KIDS AND BELIEVED WE COULD DO ANYTHING?

The saying "From the mouth of babes" is spot-on. Children don't hold back, they really live like they mean it. Case in point, an amazing story from a CanSer Cowgirl on my blog:

> My nine-year-old son and a friend were playing out front. I heard the little boy say to my son, "Your mom doesn't look very pretty without her hair." I cringed at how cruel kids can be (even without meaning to be). I had no idea what to expect from my son, until I heard his reply . . . "My mom is the most beautiful person on the earth, you are just looking in the wrong place. You have to be able to see her heart, and no one is more prettiful when you look there." That moment has gotten me through many a rough day. . . .

I wish I could be so purely eloquent. Sometimes children have the sweet voice of a sage, other times they carry daggers that we continually choose to stab ourselves with even after we've left childhood behind.

When I was a fiercely independent knotted hair unit of the 1970s, I loved nature. It was my church. I loved to look at the sun till my eyes burned. I'd singe my corneas and then immediately look at a tree or my neighbor. Purple, green, and yellow beams of light would glow around them. I knew

I was special, a chosen one, a psychic. Who else could see auras like me? I suppose anyone who blowtorched their vision could see a lot of things!

I spent every minute of the daylight exploring the world on my ribbon-flapping Huffy bike. My grandmother would light candles and say the rosary as she watched me burn down the street. "Look, *Abuela,* no hands!" I'd say. *"Aye, niña, cuidado!"* she'd bellow, followed by a string of really bad truck-driver curses in Spanish. Off I'd sail to the priest's house to steal daffodils for my mother. Looking back, I love the contrast between my terror of getting caught by a man of the cloth and the ballsy confidence that pulsed through my veins as I crawled on my stomach mini commando style.

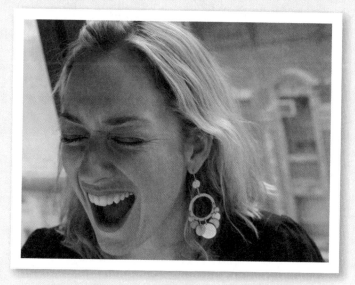

As I grew older, the doubt warts sprouted. Grown-ups, other kids, and the boob tube distorted my sense of self and occasionally made me feel handicapped. *Yes* was kidnapped by *should.* I played the recordings of mean girls on the playground in my head for decades. Why wouldn't they let me wear my Underoos in peace?

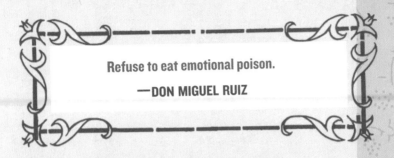

I'll never forget being tied to Britney Clowry's (name changed so that she doesn't come after me again) daily whipping post. "Kristin's so skinny she has to run around in the shower to get wet. Kristin is so ugly someone should take her down to the ASPCA and put her to sleep." The dangerous part about it was that I started to memorize that script and make it my own. Even when I was cast as the hot chick in an indie film I worried obsessively that the producers would come to their senses and fire me. A mistake must have been made. Maybe they just hired me because I was funny. The knockouts had the personality of a bag of bolts, so naturally they needed a funny girl to counterbalance the scene.

I BET YOU CAN SEE MY MADNESS CLEARLY, BUT CAN YOU SEE YOUR OWN? LET'S STOP WASTING TIME AND START FLAUNTING AND CELEBRATING OUR PRETTIFULNESS.

What were some of the **messages** you absorbed as a child?

....

....

....

....

....

....

....

....

....

....

....

....

....

....

....

....

....

....

Do you still let these descriptions define you?
Is your tattered script false and outdated?
Perhaps it's time to bring a few doubt warts to the surface
so you can slough them off . . .

....

....

....

....

....

....

....

....

....

....

....

....

....

....

....

....

....

....

....

....

....

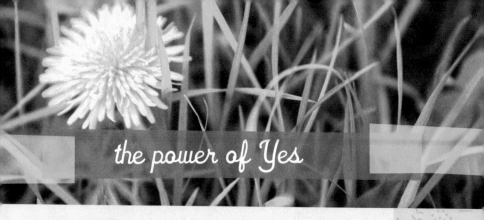

the power of Yes

What's the most powerful word in the universe?

Yes.

Some say she was the devil's spawn; others, a saint. Did she break up the Beatles? Who knows, boys will be boys and they always seem to blame it on the girls. Right? As an artist, Yoko Ono was a hoot. In 1966 she unveiled her *Ceiling Painting* at the Indica Gallery of London. Viewers had to climb up a white ladder in the center of a huge room where a magnifying glass dangled from the ceiling, allowing them to peek at an itty-bitty piece of paper with the word YES written in tiny letters and framed. It is said that that unimposing YES was almost like a whisper printed on a canvas. John and Yoko met at that exhibit. He later remarked: "It's a great relief when you get up the ladder and look through the spyglass and it doesn't say no . . . it says YES."

Yoko explained her take on the most powerful word in the universe saying, "There were many incredible negative elements in my life, and in the world, and because of that I had to conjure up a positive attitude within me in balance to the most chaotic . . . and I had to balance that by activating the 'Yes' element."

Balance out the negative elements in your own life. Post YES all over your house. Sticky notes work well. I learned this from *The Bodacious Book of Succulence: Daring to Live Your Succulent Wild Life!* by Sark. Throw it on your Crazy Sexy syllabus. It will make your chakras spin.

Affirmations

Living in the future, resisting the past, and gunning through the present. Yuck, gross. Sound familiar? That's a one-way ticket to shrivelville. Now let me lift the veil so you can see a glimpse of what I see in you. This is what your soul whispers even when your ears are too clogged to hear. Are you ready to witness the tip of the iceberg that is the glorious you? Are you ready for the truth? If you said *yes,* read on. If you said *no*—tough luck, scaredy-cat, read on anyway.

I am beautiful.

I am brilliant.

I am healthy.

I am enough.

I am wealthy.

I am empowered.

I am loved and loving.

I am forgiving and forgiven.

I am open.

I am compassionate.

I am accepting.

I am truthful.

I am supported.

I am strong.

I am blessed with a gorgeous face and body.

I am not alone.

The list is long. In the space below, please fill out the rest. If you need more space (go, lady, go!), bring this exercise into your gratitude journal. **Take ownership of your greatness—if you don't, nobody else will.**

....

....

....

....

....

....

....

....

....

....

....

You are not cancer.
You are the magnificence you just listed.

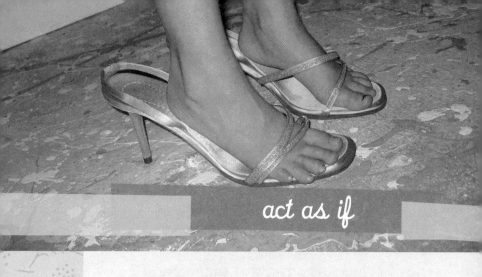

act as if

"*I'm still spinning my wheels* and stuck in the mud. What now?" You've acknowledged what you love, tapped into the hot spring of gratitude, sung your affirmations, bonfired the outdated scripts, and possibly even added a pinch of witchcraft "just in case." But for some stinking reason you still don't believe in your fabulosity. Well, I got one more trick for ya: Act as if. That's right, fake it till you make it. Attitude champs and Olympians have used this training method for generations. Catch the beam and shine it out even if you feel too dark to bathe in it. Before long you will acknowledge and accept your greatness, without apology.

Remember, we successfully manifest our dreams when the feelings behind our intentions are in alignment. Sounds simple but if you're a canSer babe it can be tough. Our stakes are higher so our fears are bigger. For example, I know that it is very important to find peace and acceptance with my diagnosis in order to live happily with cancer. But that doesn't prevent me from seeing myself as healthy and continuing to work on my recovery. I leave room for miracles and I support those potential miracles by doing the best I can to boost my immune system and heal my body. I put it out to the universe. Still, every once in a while that pesky little voice chirps, "You'll never get there, you will always be sick and you will die of cancer." Excuse me, bitch?

Do scary negative thoughts have the power to undo or sabotage all the hard work I've done? No way. If I allowed myself to believe my doubts I'd be panic struck. Every "what if" would conjure paranoid attempts to amputate my feelings in the hopes of generating signal interference. "Quick Kris, jumble your fatalistic thought waves before the universe has a chance to listen and follow suit." Talk about exhausting.

In these moments it's a good idea to turn to classic rock. Remember that bluesy song "Soulshine" by the Allman Brothers? It's a great little ditty to hum or air strum while bopping through your day.

THOSE FELLAS HAD THEIR FINGERS ON THE PULSE OF A UNIVERSAL TRUTH. SHINE IT OUT EVEN IF YA DON'T FEEL IT, ACT AS IF. LET YOUR SOUL SHINE TILL THE BREAK OF DAY.

Acting as if teaches us to believe in ourselves and to never settle for less. When weird thoughts come up we immediately correct and replace them with positive visualizations and affirmations. "My body is healthy and strong. My mind is peaceful and I am content." We catch our words and rewrite them. Confidence and self-reliance come from a deep trust in yourself. You know that you've got your back and that no matter what, you will not abandon yourself. It takes courage to build confidence. Because the only way to really do it is to put yourself out there and take risks.

I used to think it was arrogant to show my happiness—like I was bragging if I shared the good things in my life. I joined the herd and bitched with the best of them. It's just so easy to do. Politics, the environment, the economy, the war, you name it, there is plenty to complain about! Then I got slammed by Hurricane CanSer, my levees broke, and my world was drowning. In that moment I realized that the secret to happiness is the decision to be happy. Cancer is here, so now what? Fold up, Kris, or find your eagle feathers?

The Talmud says, "During the time of the darkest night, act as if the morning has already come." Fake it till you make it. Buddha (the ultimate dude) taught that the purpose of life was suffering and the end of suffering. Which to me means that when you're at your lowest, swim deeper than you've ever been willing to go, where blue becomes black. That's when you'll find a buried treasure (and a tank of oxygen).

Try on your new confidence until it fits. What's the worst thing that could happen? Nothing! Earth to you, come in you: The worst (and best) that can happen already has! You have nothing to lose.

For more on the topic of personal transformation, immediately read anything by Marianne Williamson.

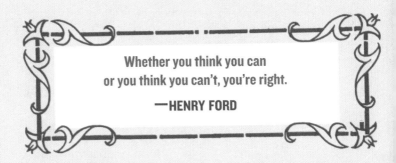

Whether you think you can
or you think you can't, you're right.
—HENRY FORD

Make believe time!

What does the woman or man you desire to become look like? How does she act? Dress? Speak? What aspects of yourself would need to change in order to become more like her? Don't be stingy with the details.

HAVE FUN AND DELVE INTO YOUR IMAGINATION.

....

....

....

....

....

....

....

....

....

....

....

....

....

....

....

....

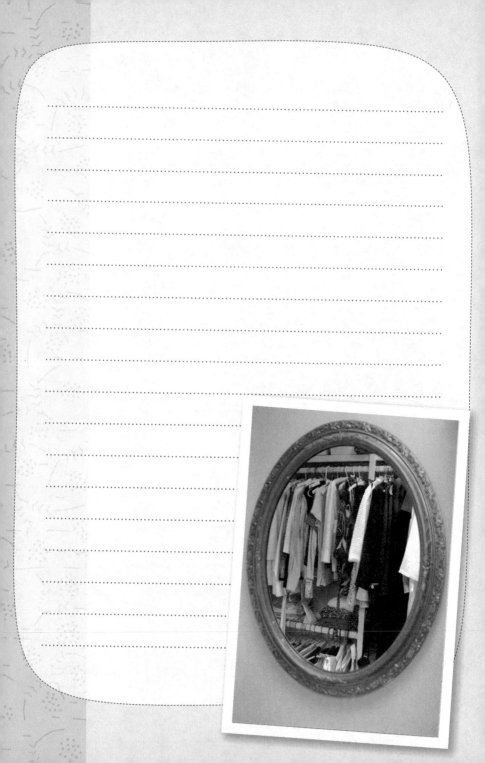

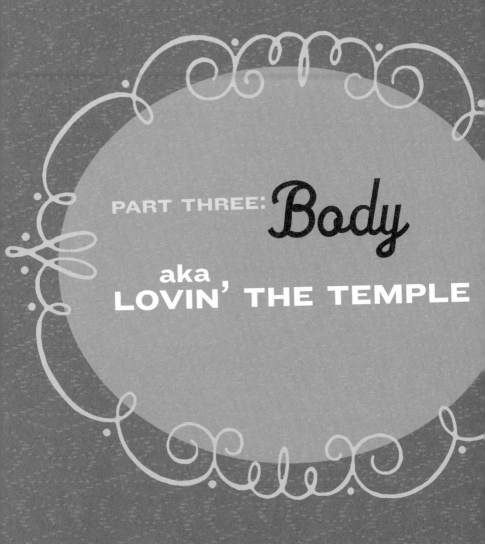

PART THREE: *Body*

aka,
LOVIN' THE TEMPLE

One of my teachers once asked, "Out of diet, exercise, and meditation, which helps you heal the most?" I thought diet—healthy chow has always been my sun and my moon.

Then she gave us the answer: "The one you're not doing." Brain explosion!

I'm a layperson, an educated civilian with no special degrees from Ivy League houses. I'm not a professional in any body modalities—not in nutrition, exercise, beauty, massage, any of the myriad ways we CanSer Cowgirls and dudes can hasten our healing. What I *do* have, though, is experience—lots of years using and abusing and celebrating this imperfect-getting-perfect body. In this part of the book, I'll share with you what I've learned along my long, long adventure, from more ways your thoughts change your health to the best stuff to put on, and in, your body. If you're at all interested, please do your research, experiment, and find the path that works for you. And never stop exploring!

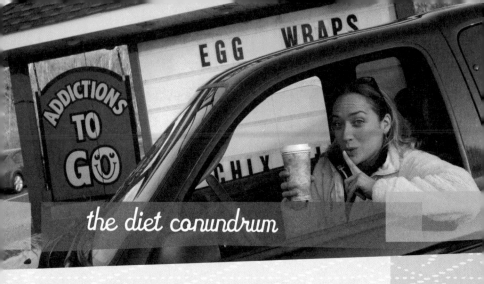

the diet conundrum

What should I eat? Healthy or sick, it's a question that plagues us all. It's so confusing, and fad diets and best seller lists pull us in different directions. Why doesn't one diet just take care of it all? Instead of looking directly at the picture, look at the negative space around it. The one thing most reputable diets have in common isn't what they tell you to eat, it's what they tell you *not* to eat.

The body is phenomenally mysterious, and yet the answer to the diet conundrum is actually quite straight-forward: Eat food. "Well of course I eat food," you say. But do you? Food isn't made in a laboratory. Food comes from nature, from the garden. Food is easily pronounced and doesn't come with warning labels. When we make the connection between what we consume and how we feel, a great transformational shift can occur. I've said it before, I'll say it again: No one knows more about you than you. Really listen to what your body is telling you. She does speak, but you have to *fermez la bouche* (that's "shut up" in French—sounds more polite) so you can hear her!

Lots of folks ask me what I eat. Here goes: I am a vegan and I follow a mostly raw-food diet. But I must say it took a lot of transitioning to get to a place where basic foods felt really satisfying. In the beginning I experienced many detox symptoms and sugar cravings. Over time I have learned how to set a doable pace for changing my diet and upgrading my lifestyle. Now I thoroughly enjoy my healthy diet. My average day is pretty simple. I start each day with a cup or two of warm water with lemon (highly alkalizing and flushes the liver), followed by 16 to 32 ounces of freshly juiced greens and veggies. This usually holds me till noon. After that 70 to 80 percent of each meal is raw, while the remaining 20 to 30 percent is cooked and properly combined. (For more on food combining, read the nutrition chapter in *Crazy Sexy Cancer Tips.*) You may need more food or find a better combination for your lifestyle needs.

Look at your plate and break it down like a pie. The vast majority of space should be taken up by fresh and organic salads and veggies. Make sense? Follow this ratio to better health, but start slowly. Maybe 50/50 is where you need to be at first. Or, if you are in a healing crisis, perhaps 100 percent raw is best for you. Since I changed the way I eat post-diagnosis, I have seen massive improvements in my overall health. That doesn't mean I'm "cured" but it does mean I feel much better. It's important to do your homework and understand how to eat this way. You can be what I call a "muffin vegetarian" and still feel pretty tired and lousy. In my experience, a vibrant and effective vegan or vegetarian diet means that the majority of your food comes from vegetables!

Remember high school science class? Well, if you don't, here's a little refresher course. The body maintains a delicate pH balance. Neutral pH is 7. The higher the pH (greater than 7) the more alkaline; while a pH lower than 7 is acidic. For good health our bodies need to be slightly alkaline (with a pH of between 7.365 and 7.45). By eating a more alkaline diet (leafy greens, wheatgrass, veggies, sprouts, juicing) as opposed to an acidic diet (high in animal products, processed foods, sugar, and starch), we flood our bodies with oxygen, enzymes, vitamins, minerals, and chlorophyll. Chlorophyll contains a powerful blood builder that's said to

increase red blood cells, improve circulation, ease inflam-
mation, oxygenate the body, and counteract harmful free
radicals. By eating a diet high in chlorophyll we dine on
liquid oxygen and sunlight. Mama Earth helps us to thrive
and heal our bodies.

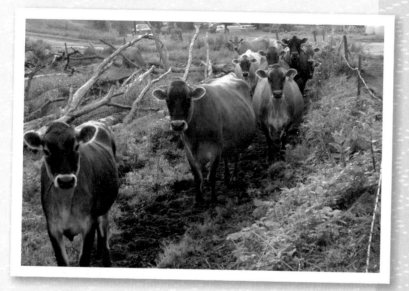

Healthy food creates healthy cells and healthy thoughts.
Conversely, junk goes in and junk comes out. If it's invented
in a laboratory, it'll take a laboratory to digest it. If it has
a shelf life longer than yours, wake up, don't eat it! Look at
your plate, peek in your glass. What direction are you moving in? On the pH scale, Soda = 2. Coffee = 4. Cucumber = 7.
Get the picture? Burger, fries, Diet Coke, muffin, candy bar,
booze? Acid bath! Green drinks, salads, sprouts, wheatgrass?
Alkaline super disco! Your goal is to make energy deposits
instead of constant withdrawals.

One of the biggest causalities of the SAD—standard
American diet—is the toll it takes on the body, especially
the digestive system, liver, and kidneys. When we feed our
bodies nutrient-deficient foods, we exhaust our enzymatic
reserves and mine minerals like potassium, calcium, and

magnesium from our bones, teeth, and organs to neutralize the acids. We create free radicals that damage our cells and rob electrons from healthy tissue. As a result, our system weakens and basic functions begin to break down. In a nutshell, I have just described the aging process. It is also a fertile ground for the seeds of degenerative illnesses. How can we press stop, rewind, and restart? Pull a garbage can up to your fridge and cupboards and treat yourself to a lifestyle makeover!

Many people have chewed and sipped their way to being cancer-free after adopting a vegan/vegetarian diet consisting of 70 to 100 percent raw foods with the emphasis on vegetables, some fruits, seeds, nuts, seaweeds, and daily juicing. Whether it will happen for you (or me), I cannot promise. But one thing I know for certain: Other physical ailments will vanish. You will feel fantastic energy and you will strengthen your immune system. Aches, pains, high blood pressure, elevated cholesterol, sinus and allergy problems, constipation, fatigue, and even arthritis and other degenerative diseases can all be reversed. Your skin will clear up and your breath will be sweet. You can slow the aging process. Whoa, now I've got your attention!

Raw foods clear a path for regeneration, but healing takes time, and at first we may find it difficult. When peristalsis (the contraction of smooth muscles that propels stuff through the digestive tract) is weak, stagnation backs up our delicate system. Waste pollutes our body and fogs our thinking. The introduction of a better diet loaded with fiber kicks our lazy and aloof intestines into high gear. It's like taking a junk-food sloth to the gym and expecting him to bench press his own weight on day one. Oftentimes, the more sick a person is, the more taxed their digestive system has become.

Enter juicing! By removing the fiber through the process of squeezing the pulp, we instantly lighten our digestive load. Nutrients pass directly into the bloodstream, and within minutes our bodies receive optimum fuel to feed our cells and help restore our immune systems. This doesn't mean we don't eat certain sprouted and cooked grains, salads, and other intestinal brooms—we do. If you follow these dietary guidelines you will get plenty of fiber. However, juicing gives our bodies a much needed rest and boosts our pH. It's a critical part of our healing game plan. If our bodies spend less energy on digestion, they will spend more on repair. Smoothies are great too, but remember, smoothies have fiber. Love them, make them, rely on them for a change, but make sure that juice is your staple.

Dr. Ginger and I spend many hours on the phone gabbing about diet, changing the world, and race car drivers. It's really important to have and make friends who are into the same revolutionary ideas as you. Ginger and I constantly educate ourselves in order to share what we've learned with our friends and family. After one of our powwows, I asked her to write an article for this book. The guidelines I gave were simple: "The title is Fight Cancer with Your Fork. Go for it." If food is your passion and you believe that knowledge is power, read the next section with an open and curious mind. Thank you, Ginger, my wonderful teacher!

Fight Cancer with Your Fork

Despite what your doc may tell you, there are plenty of things you can do to take control of your health destiny. Right after ridding yourself of all mental constipation by putting your mind in the right space for healing, your fork is your next best anti-cancer defense weapon.

Here is my list of top strategies to get your immune system hummin' "Happy Days Are Here Again." These may be big chow changes for many of you, so if you're not ready to fully loosen your grip on your standard American diet (SAD) vittles, simply pick out a few from the list to get rolling. And remember, your body is constantly churning over new cells. If the building blocks for those new cells are garbage, you will by default only produce garbage cells.

Here are some of the bad apples to keep out of
your healthy, cancer-free kitchen:

No-no 1:

Caffeine. Caffeine is in reality a legal drug, and
like many drugs it can become highly addictive.
If you've ever quit your morning cup-o'-joe cold
turkey and experienced those mind-blowing with-
drawal headaches, you know what I mean. *You*
need to be in control of your body, not some drug
in your grub. Eliminate coffee, soda, diet soda,
energy drinks, caffeinated water, and caffeinated
teas, including black, green, and oolong teas. Also,
no "decaffeinated" teas; they can still amp you up.
Most still have some caffeine left in them, as well
as solvent residues from the chemical decaffeina-
tion process. Consume only teas that are naturally
decaffeinated and organic. Go get wired from
green juices instead, and remember that chocolate
also contains caffeine (and dairy).

No-no 2:

**Processed, packaged, refined, canned, micro-
wavable, non-organic or frozen foods.** Eliminate
bagels, unsprouted breads, cakes, candy bars, cere-
als, fried and processed chips, conventional condi-
ments, cookies, crackers, jellies, jams, microwave
popcorn (air pop instead), canned and roasted
nuts (raw nuts only), white pretzels, processed
granola/trail mix, protein bars (unless they're
raw), store-bought salad dressings, conventional
jarred sauces and dips, packaged or canned soups,
toaster pastries, and TV dinners. This includes *all*
"diet" products: diet shakes and sodas, diet frozen
TV dinners, and anything labeled "sugar-free,"
"fat-free," or "light." Have you read or even tried
to pronounce the ingredients in these things? Also
avoid processed whey, casein or soy protein powders, and anything made with white sugar, white
flour, white rice, and white table salt. Yes, this is a

long list (and I'm sure I've left out a few things). It may, in fact, be all the foods you currently eat, but these foods are highly processed, nutrient-defunct, acidic, and toxic, and they do nothing but *take away* from your health. As ninety-four-year-old fitness guru Jack LaLanne says, "If man made it, don't eat it." Live by that motto.

No-no 3:

Animal products. As if number 2 wasn't shocking enough, yep, elimination of acidic animal protein is another golden nugget in the treasure chest of radical reversal and prevention of diseases, including cancer. I recommend that you read *The China Study*, by T. Colin Campbell, to understand and drive home the many reasons why it is so important to eliminate animal protein. Here's one for ya: Studies have shown that animal protein accelerates cancer's growth. This is one reason why many healing centers around the world, like the Hippocrates Health Institute, immediately ban all animal products from their clients' diets. So forgo meat of any kind: beef, chicken, turkey, wild game, all fish including shellfish and sushi, and all processed deli meats, hot dogs, and prepackaged meats. In addition, cut out dairy, including butter, margarine spreads, cheese, cream cheese, yogurt, milk, and ice cream. Eliminate eggs, including egg whites and egg substitutes. The bottom-line philosophy: Don't eat anything with a face, a liver, or a mother.

No-no 4:

Artificial sweeteners. Many have said that artificial sweeteners should be added to the FDA's Hall of Shame, for they are potent nerve toxins and never should have been approved as safe for human consumption. They have the potential to freak out and damage your nervous system— your brain and nerves—leading to a variety of symptoms from migraine headaches to unexplained seizures, dizziness, depression, and vision problems. There are even links to cancer, obesity, and diabetes. I bet you didn't realize how many of these human-made tasty toxins you gobble up on a daily basis. They hide out in thousands of your favorite foods, including diet meals, flavored waters, popular drink mixes such as Crystal Light, many commercial salad dressings, and—ready for this?—even over-the-counter medicines like Alka-Seltzer, toothpastes, gum, vitamins, and those Listerine breath strips! The use of chemical sweeteners of *any* kind—aspartame, NutraSweet, Equal, Sweet'N Low, saccharin, Canderel, and even Splenda—is not advised. Don't go there. And don't be duped by their sugarcoated advertising. The commercials may say, "Tastes like sugar because it's made from sugar," but that particular product is highly processed and has been laced with chlorine. And get this: Sugar is not even one of the ingredients on its product label! Huh? The answer: raw organic agave or, even better, stevia. Both can be picked up at your local health food store.

No-no 5:

Soy. Okay, close your gaping mouth. I know, you thought soy was a health food—after all, that's what is plastered all over every media outlet. Keep in mind that Big Food makes big bucks from advertising their highly processed (and oftentimes genetically modified) soy milk, soy cheese, soy ice cream, soy chips, and soy protein bars as "health" foods. There are so many of these foods on the market today, you literally could go through an entire day and eat nothing but highly processed soy products. Here's the deal: The studies performed on Asian communities showing the positive health benefits of soy involved *fermented* soy products, like tempeh, miso, and natto (foods most people in this country have never even heard of, much less eaten), in *condiment* portions. Get it? That's *fermented soy in condiment portions*. A far cry from the fake health foods made with preservatives and other chemicals advertised ad nauseam as cure-alls that are consumed by unsuspecting consumers in this country. Don't be bamboozled!

Chow time! Bust a grub on all these good eats *every single day:*

tip 1:

Drink green juice *daily*. Nothing is going to send those cancer devils to their death more effectively than boosting your immune system by saturating your body with fresh-made, organic, raw green juices and green smoothies. It's like opening a big

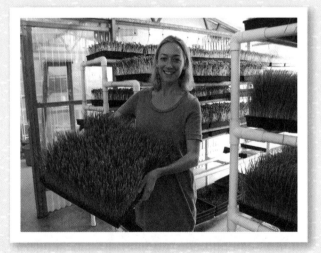

can of whoop-ass. Utilize your basic organic green veggies such as cucumber and celery, add some dark leafy greens and cruciferous vegetables, throw in some pea and sunflower sprouts, and even work a few ounces of wheatgrass into your daily routine. Not only will you be amazed at the highly charged energy you have, but your body will be thanking you for the super-nourishment, the balancing of blood sugars, the plant protein, and the loads of toxins being purged from their hiding places. Consume a *minimum* of thirty-six ounces of green juice per day. Oh, and store-bought juices don't count; they are not raw, unless they are made fresh in front of you.

Note: Consult your doctor if you are taking blood thinners such as Coumadin (warfarin) before green juicing. Ironically, you will be instructed not to consume healthy greens or life-giving green veggie juices. When you're consuming a healthy diet of greens such as broccoli, kale, spinach, and collard greens, ingestion of a variety of nutrients with vitamins E and K naturally balances the blood-clotting mechanisms so you don't bleed to death or, conversely, develop a deadly clot. But if you are prescribed blood-thinning medications, you are usually firmly instructed by your doctor to avoid all greens and green juices: The vitamin K in greens decreases the effectiveness of the drug, so you will need more medication. Blood thinners are a very dangerous class of medications and must be monitored very closely with frequent, often weekly, blood tests. *You cannot stop taking blood thinners or alter the doses yourself without working with your doctor, or you will risk bleeding to death.* Some

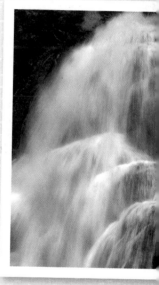

doctors will work closely with you on your drug doses while you eat greens, as long as the amount of vitamin K from greens consumed is consistent each day; others will forbid all greens, and still others will forgo blood thinners altogether and balance blood-clotting abilities through foods and supplements containing vitamins K and E. Find a doctor who will work with your choice.

tip 2:

Eat real food. Chomp only on a variety of *real* food: fresh, raw, organic whole fruits, vegetables, and soaked nuts and seeds. Don't let this short list deceive you. There are hundreds of choices within these food categories and literally thousands of tasty recipes you can make with nature's chow.

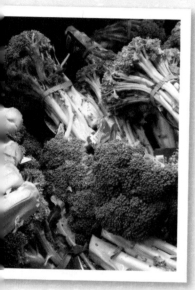

In particular, focus on vegetable juices, dark leafy greens, cruciferous veggies, sea vegetables (dulse, kelp, nori, arame, and so on), and loads of sprouts—which are cheap and very easy to grow yourself. These are highly nutritious, alkaline plant proteins that will throw your healing gear into full throttle and your nutritional deficiencies out the window.

Note: Limit sweet fruit while you're healing from cancer, diabetes, or bacterial and yeast infections. Modern fruit is so hybridized, it is estimated to be up to thirty times sweeter than wild, natural fruit. The human body was not meant to handle this volume of sugar, especially when battling a health challenge.

tip 3:

Add more raw food. When you cook your food, you literally cook the life and the "magic" out of it—

and dangerous, toxic carcinogens in. So eat almost all, if not all, of your food in its natural, raw form. Eating raw ensures that you get the food's mother lode of oxygen, chlorophyll, and alkaline nutrients (all destroyed in cooking) and none of the nasty toxins—like acrylamides, heterocyclic amines, or free radicals—that are produced by cooking. Pick up a raw-food recipe book to learn how to make pasta, pizza, and even yumptious desserts using only plant protein: fruits, veggies, nuts, and seeds. Your temple will bow in praise.

tip 4:

Drink clean, filtered water. Clean, filtered water is essential to good health but darn hard to find, for it doesn't just stream right out of the tap that way these days. Common toxins such as chlorine (which kills off the good bacteria in your intestines and creates cancer-causing agents when it comes into contact with organic material already present in the water) and fluoride (which causes fluorosis, or mottling of the tooth enamel, and has been linked to thyroid dysfunction) abound. Other not-so-well-known nasty carcinogenic toxins such as industrial contaminants, heavy metals, pesticides, rocket fuel, and factory farm wastes discharged into streams and rivers are also finding their way into our drinking water. Even prescription meds flushed down the toilet and toxic personal body care products washed away in the shower have been detected in our municipal water. According to the Environmental Working Group's (www.ewg.org) National Assessment of Tap Water Quality Report of 2005, 260 contaminants were found in our nation's tap water (and this was only what was tested for), more than half of which have no health-based safety standards *whatsoever*. You can lessen what's lurking in your water by consuming only water that has been filtered. Keep in mind that you want to think about bathing, showering, and swimming in filtered water, too, as your skin is your body's large absorptive (and eliminative) organ, so everything that touches it is absorbed. Rinse your fruits and veggies and soak your nuts and seeds in filtered water as well.

tip 5:

Take food-based supplements daily. Although it is estimated that about 70 percent of adults use supplements, with at least 50 percent of those using a general multivitamin, I totally agree with Kris when she says, "Supplements are just that, supplements to our diet, not the main course."

You should derive most of your nutrients from organic, raw, whole food, but keep in mind that our water, air, and entire environment are more toxic today than ever before and our produce, due to chemically depleted soil, is also nutritionally inferior. Processing, storage, and cooking of food significantly deplete vital nutrients as well, so in addition to eating more raw, organic, uncooked food, some basic supplements are in order for most.

It might surprise you to know that not all vitamin supplements are created equal. There are essentially two kinds: synthetic, chemical supplements and whole-food supplements.

Whole-food supplements are food concentrates made by taking nature's bounty of organically grown whole foods, drying them in a dehydrator, grinding them up into powders, and then encapsulating or compressing them into pills or tablets. As with organic, raw whole foods like fruits and veggies, whole-food supplements have a very complex bundle of "living" nutrients, phytochemicals, bioflavonoids, enzymes, co-enzymes, and thousands of other *plant* chemicals yet to be discovered by scientists that must work synergistically together to produce their "magic" in your body.

Synthetic, chemical supplements, on the other hand, are isolated chemical compounds created by a pharmaceutical scientist in a lab. "Let's put some vitamin A, B, C, D, E, and K together with some minerals and voilà, we have a best-selling supplement to be taken once a day by millions and can be sold at every grocery store, wholesale club, and corner pharmacy." Nature, however, doesn't work that way. Studies in journals such as *The American Journal of Clinical Nutrition, Annals of the New York Academy of Sciences,* and publications of the Royal Society of Chemistry show that nutrients in isolation are not utilized properly by the body. Both nutrient integrity and bioavailability is lacking in "dead," synthetic, chemical supplements. You can't just pop an isolated synthetic nutrient and expect it to work like Mother Nature. As Dr. T. Colin Campbell, professor emeritus of nutrition at Cornell University, says, "Isolating nutrients and trying to get the benefits equal to those in whole foods reveals an ignorance of how nutrition operates in the body."

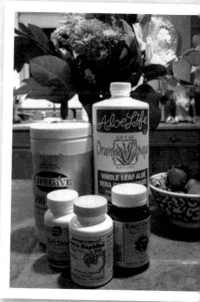

For example, scurvy, the classic sailor's disease caused by a deficiency of vitamin C, cannot be cured by taking chemically synthesized ascorbic acid, the isolated nutrient found in many popular synthetic vitamin C tablets. To prevent or reverse scurvy, you need additional plant compounds like quercetin, rutin, bioflavonoids, and many other phytochemicals.

Synthetic, chemical supplements are in fact quite toxic to the body. Some manufacturers of soft gel supplements use hydrogenated oils (trans fats)—including partially hydrogenated soybean oils—as fillers. This makes no sense to me. How can a company selling a supplement touted as good for health be using a commonly known toxic ingredient? Even the National Academy of Sciences states that there is *no* safe level of trans fat intake.

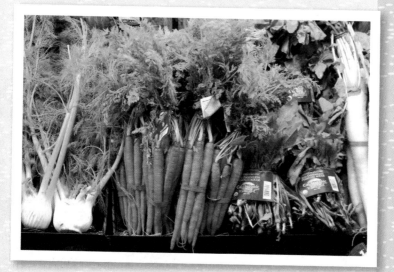

Make sure your daily multivitamin says "whole-food supplement" on the label.

Here are some other food-based basic supplements to have in your arsenal:

- Digestive enzymes.
- Superfoods like chlorella and blue-green algae.
- Probiotics.
- Vitamin B12.
- Organic green powders. (Great for travel!)

Work with a holistic doctor on other items you may need for your specific health challenges.

"Worst, Better, Best"

If you now feel like you are drowning in the Nutritional Bermuda Triangle, let me throw you a great big life preserver to help you ride the current and stay afloat: These changes don't all have to be made overnight, although if you are facing a serious health challenge, you may want to step up the pace . . . pretty quickly. It takes more intensity and effort to reverse a disease than to prevent one. In the end, it is essential to have a new relationship with food and to eat as cleanly as possible if you hope to give your temple all the tools and fuels it needs to put your condition into reverse and stay super healthy. There is, however, a way to tiptoe into it, if you will.

I call it "Worst, Better, Best Transitioning." It involves transitioning from the worst choice in a category of food to the better choice, and then to the best. If you are ready to move from worst to best right away, a big high five to you, but if you're not, this can be a great way to ease yourself in. If you are presently eating in the better food categories, it's time *right now* to hightail yourself into the best. One thing *everyone* should be doing is green juicing every day!

Here are some more tips to make your ride to heavenly health a little smoother:

tip 1:

Get off caffeine. Coffee, soda, and energy drinks are in the worst category, no doubt about it. You can wean yourself off them by consuming green tea, which I consider a better caffeine source. The best, of course, is to be on your own natural high

If you really think about the foods you consume, I bet you can envision for yourself what the "worst, better, best" choices would be for a particular selection.

HERE'S YOUR ASSIGNMENT:

Make a list of ten foods you want to transition into and list their worst, better, and best versions. Don't hang out in the worst or better categories for a long period of time. Plan the time frame of your smooth move into the best categories—and watch your health rock!

	FOOD NAME	WORST	BETTER	BEST
1				
2				
3				
4				
5				
6				
7				
8				
9				
10				

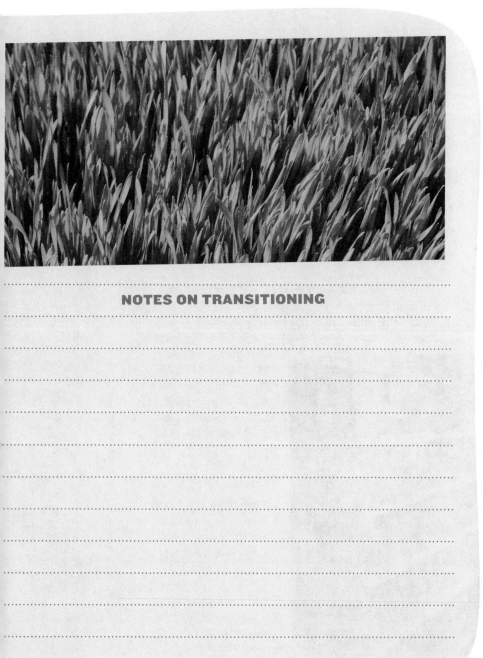

NOTES ON TRANSITIONING

and consume *no* caffeine, especially if a health challenge is looking you square in the face. Turn your green juice into your new coffee in the morning and throughout the day. Here is what one client of mine said: "I really love the stimulation I get from the [green] drink. You were right, it is ten times better than caffeine."

tip 2:

Improve your pasta. Regular pasta made from white flour with a store-bought traditional marinara sauce is the worst choice when it comes to pasta. The better choice would be an organic quinoa (pronounced *KEEN-wah*) pasta (no gluten, no pesticides) and an organic jarred pasta sauce (with no cheese) from your local health food store. But the absolute healthiest option is a raw pasta made from zucchini in a spiralizer or Saladacco, served with raw marinara sauce and topped with

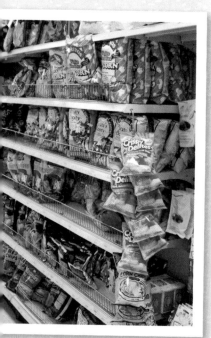

a raw-nut cheese (you can mix this up in no time in a blender). *Yum!* This dish also doesn't make you feel like you need to sleep for a week after you eat.

tip 3:

The chips are down. Regular potato chips are the worst. Health-food-store-bought veggie chips are better—although they still use canola oil and contain acrylamides and other toxic by-products of cooking. Veggie chips sprinkled with cayenne pepper and sea vegetables like dulse and kelp made in a dehydrator are totally best.

tip 4:

Find better meat, chicken, and fish choices. If you insist on eating animal products, at the very least make sure they are organic. This ensures that they are free of antibiotics and hormones. Still, remember that these are animal products, which are not healing foods. The best choice, of course, is a plant-protein-based diet, especially for those with cancer.

tip 5:

There *is* a better chocolate. Regular milk chocolate, as in a candy bar or chocolate syrup, is in the worst category. Raw cacao is better (if it's not made with milk), and raw carob (which has no dairy *or* caffeine) is the best.

Isn't Dr. Ginger cool? I'm lucky she joined my posse. It's important to understand what food does for and to your body. But as Dr. Ginger says, don't expect massive changes overnight. Baby steps. Remember, think *transition,* not *perfection.* This is about improving your life, not ruining it. The stress of change can be just as acidic as a hunk of milk chocolate–coated no-no. The goal is healthy cells and we need to do our best to put one foot in front of the other in order to break our old patterns and reach our end point: health. You are on the train. Some days you are the conductor, other days you hang on to the caboose. But guess what? We're all on the 5:08 and by God we're moving forward. Life is sweet. Enjoy the process of waking up.

FIND YOUR JOY AND KNOW THAT YOU ARE A WHITE LIGHT DISCO WITH NO CEILINGS AND NO LIMITATIONS. NOW GO MAKE A SALAD.

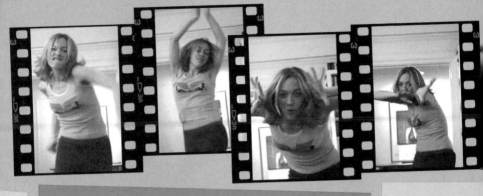

shake your ass!

Exercise floods the body with oxygen and rids it of toxins via the lymphatic system. The body has two circulatory systems, one for blood and the other for lymph (a colorless fluid that bathes every cell in the body). The blood is lucky: It gets circulated by that pump called the heart. Lymph, on the other hand, is circulated by a pump called exercise. Many tissues depend on lymph to provide nutrients (including oxygen) and carry off wastes. If the lymph doesn't circulate, then the tissues suffocate by sitting in the stagnation of their own acidic waste products.

One of the best ways to exercise is to jump on a mini trampoline or rebounder. As you bounce, your cells get gently squeezed by the alternation of weightlessness and gravitational pull. As a result, toxins are flushed and nutrition floods your body. It's also extremely gentle on your joints. If you're too wiped out to jump, then sit and bounce or do gentle stretches. Light movement is better than no movement at all.

I can recommend lots of different types of exercise, everything from yoga (my personal favorite) to karate. But the best kind is the kind you'll actually do. So figure out what you like best and get moving!

LET'S FACE IT, BESIDES THE PHYSICAL BENEFITS IT DELIVERS, EXERCISE JUST MAKES YOU FEEL GOOD.

Exercise releases endorphins and is a great overall attitude adjuster. Experts suggest we get our hearts pumping three to five times a week for about thirty-five minutes.

Add some weight training to that and you're protecting yourself from bone loss. Yup, did you know that weight-bearing exercise is one of the best ways to fend off osteoporosis, especially once you cut back on or give up the cow juice? So get out there and shake your ass, do some Down Dogs, buy a hula hoop, round up your posse and practice double Dutch, or hit the streets or fields for a brisk walk, gentle trot, or all-out run. You're a warrior, so start your training. If you're stuck in a hospital bed or extremely debilitated (for now), don't fret. Try some restorative yoga, connect with a physical therapist, practice deep cleansing breaths. Visualize yourself shaking your booty and healing your temple! Never underestimate the mind–body connection.

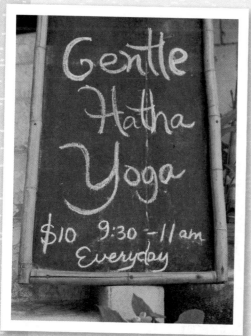

WRITE DOWN the types of exercise that you enjoy (and will do).
When and where can you do them?
What are the obstacles that make this hard and how can you overcome them?

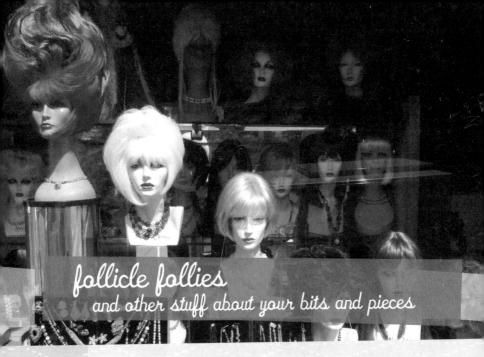

follicle follies
and other stuff about your bits and pieces

What's your real expression of power? Is it your hair, those long locks that signify your femininity? Is it a midriff that exposes a toned and scar-free body? A nice rack and a tight tush? That's the easy answer. You can purchase that stuff. Your real expression of power will come when you stop forcing yourself into a box and start speaking your well-informed mind. My power is my pen. Think about those geriatric male rock stars who continue to strut around like they're all that and a bag of chips. Lots of those fellas are tough on the eyes, but there's still something about them that makes your kitten purr. That something is the unwavering belief in self.

Cancer pushes all our insecurities to the surface. The first thing I asked when I was diagnosed was, "Will I lose my hair?" The second question was "Will I die?"—second! That's how important my hair was to me. As it turned out, my follicles stayed untouched but my self-confidence plummeted. I still recognized the girl in the mirror, but I sensed that a part of her had gone missing. I wanted to stick a picture of myself on a milk carton and hope that someone would relocate me intact. Excuse me waitress, can I have a reality check?

In a recent article about the grande dame of the feminist movement, Gloria Steinem, the former undercover Playboy Bunny talked about the process of aging. She described getting older as a freeing and empowering experience. "In a general way, women become more radical as they get older. The pattern is that women are conservative when they're young. That's when there's the most pressure on us to conform, when we're potential child bearers and sex objects." Steinem went on to say that she wished that she had been more compassionate with herself. She wished that our future selves could meet our past selves and tell them, "It's OK, it's OK." The feisty 71-year-old had some thunderous advice for young women today, "Do whatever they fucking well please." Ha!

Compare the process of aging to the process of recovery.

AGING GRACEFULLY DOESN'T MEAN POLITELY CASTRATING YOURSELF SO YOU CAN GO OUT WITH DIGNITY.

I want to age and heal like Gloria, to wear aviator glasses into my seventies, to paint my nails and allow them to chip, to swear and push buttons. I want to change the way people label themselves and others. Let canSer allow you to march on your inner Washington. Do it! Be radical. Safe makes me yawn.

**How do you feel about losing your
hair or any other bits and pieces?**
*Are you allowing your femininity
to be defined by your parts?*

....
....
....
....
....
....
....
....
....
....
....
....
....
....
....
....

bite your inner bitch

. . . Yup, even if you're a vegetarian. Your inner bitch is the negative voice telling you that you'll always be sick, fat, stupid, or ugly. Puncture her with your teeth and visualize the wench deflating like a balloon and flying away with fart sounds.

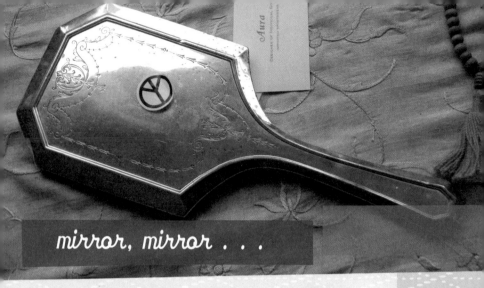

mirror, mirror . . .

Bob Dylan once said, "Being noticed can be a burden. Jesus got himself crucified because he got himself noticed. So I disappear a lot." I love this quote for so many reasons. Dylan could easily be describing how a CanSer Cowgirl feels on an oh-just-fuck-it-all day. Like it or not, there are many visual clues that point out an illness. Changes in your appearance force you to wear the scarlet letter C on your sleeve. Throughout the course of this book, I have shared many of the techniques I use to diminish cancer's power. But once again, please do not assume that I don't have bad days, too. I do. I just rally the inner troops, focus on the positive, and get on with it already. The surreal trip on the disoriented express will take you to moments when the only action you can muster is to fade. This road is long and hard, and disappearing can seem like a very appealing vacation from it all. But as with all vacations, you eventually must go home and face the music.

SOMETIMES NO MATTER HOW MUCH YOU KNOW YOU SHOULD FOCUS ON YOUR INNER BEAUTY, YOU JUST CAN'T GET PAST WHAT YOU SEE ON THE OUTSIDE.

When you look in the mirror and freak out about what cancer has taken from you, there is only one thing left to do. Tap into your inner Madonna! Remember when Madonna performed "Like a Virgin" at the MTV Video Music Awards in the early 1980s? As she writhed around the floor in a white wedding dress and plastic bangles, my world stood still. This was a whole lotta woman exploding before my thirteen-year-old eyes. Madonna rocketed to mega-goddess status for one very important reason. She constantly reinvented herself.

Take a page from Madonna's playbook and get yourself a new look. Go through your closet and toss what isn't you right now. A good rule of thumb is that if you haven't worn it in the past year, you won't wear it in the next one. Clutter makes my head explode; I need room for the new me to develop. The new me has style. You don't need much—a few simple and versatile pieces will do. Take risks and have fun!

Madame X

My junior year in college, I had a wicked badass nun as my art history teacher. She was supreme. Instead of hitting us with boring books, she'd send us to a museum for a million hours. "Come back with details or don't come back at all," she'd holler. On one particular crusade to the Metropolitan Museum of Art, I saw a painting that opened my eyes to a new kind of power beauty, and it changed the way I saw my distinguished profile (aka schnozz). All alone in a stairwell stood a towering, handsome woman called *Madame X* by John Singer Sargent. This lady was smokin'; she was a proud revolutionary. Critics raked her over the coals for being bold and brazen. Plus she was a bit slutty for the times, letting the strap of her evening gown hang off her shoulder. Oh, the horror. Talk about pushing boundaries and not giving a crap! I fell in love with her, my first girl crush. After my affair with the Madame I went bonkers for Frida Kahlo,

What can you get rid of? How can you update your look to add some pizzazz to your style?

REINVENT YOURSELF—
HOW DOES THE NEW YOU LOOK?

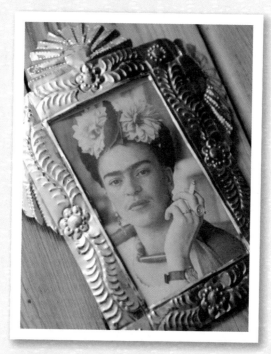

mustache and all, especially when she wore fruit and flowers in her hair and smoked filterless cigs. What a tamale! I wanted to be like *these* women, to be different and beautiful from the inside out.

You've heard this before, but I swear it's true: The most beautiful asset a woman can possess isn't her hair, her breasts, her soft skin, or her curvy hips, it's her imperfections. Think of the sexy, not-so-classic beauties who work their uniqueness, transforming it into success.

Find a new role model. Look beyond the mirror into the deep and soulful goddess you've become. You may be banged up and feeling like fifty cents rather than a million bucks, but remember, this body of yours is only a temporary house built to protect the righteous Aphrodite within. Worship her.

Name a few *unique beauties* who inspire you to dare to be different.

....
....
....
....
....
....
....
....
....
....
....
....
....
....
....
....

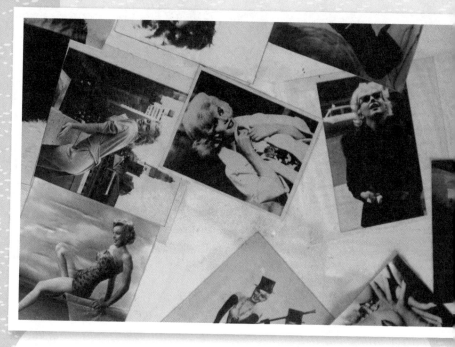

....

....

....

....

....

....

....

....

....

....

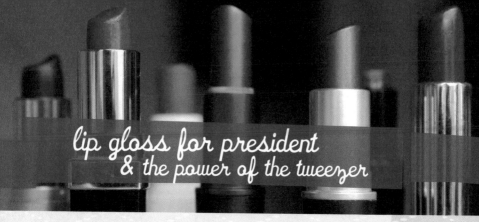

Meeting your inner beauty will be one of the best days of your life. But that doesn't mean you can't wear a little lipstick for the occasion. Sometimes concealer and a tube of gloss can kick your confidence up a notch. We're all so offended by construction-worker catcalls, but it's even more offensive when they stop. You just may need a little buffing to make you feel like you're still in the game. Here's some advice that will keep the dogs howling and resurrect your shine: Go get your hair styled, your face sparkled, and throw in a mani and a pedi for good measure.

JUST BECAUSE WE'RE SICK DOESN'T MEAN WE HAVE TO LOOK IT!

Since you are now Madonna, you need a makeup artist for your tour. Enter my friend Ann. Ann and I have known each other since we were teenagers in ballet school. I was the rebel, Ann was the swan. My mom was thrilled that such opposites could become pals. Ann's mom was horrified. Her years of proper child rearing were at risk under my troublemaking influence. Post-tutus, Ann and I would spend hours reading magazines and playing with makeup. Well, actually she was the one playing with the makeup, I was in the kitchen weighing chicken breasts on a scale and experimenting with pseudo-healthy recipes and vats of fat-free frozen yogurt from Carvel. Today Ann still plays with paint and products, but now she gets paid loads of money for it as a successful makeup artist in New York. Take it away, Ann!

Rejuvenate, Recharge, Maintain

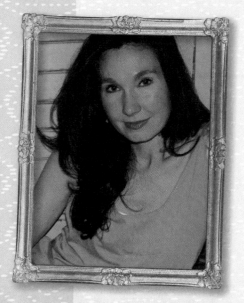

tip 1:

It's tub time. One of my favorite pick-me-ups to start my day or relax me before bed is to take a bath with either Jason Natural's body wash or Dr. Bronner's pure glycerin soap and a natural sponge. Find a fragrance that is uplifting for you—vanilla, rose, lavender, apricot, what have you. Light a candle and create a bathroom sanctuary.

tip 2:

Mask it. Take fifteen minutes, screen your calls, and hang out in a cozy robe. Flip through magazines and spend some girl time with yourself. Apply a gentle clay, hydrating, or enzyme mask to freshen your skin. Astara and Zia are two brands whose lines include natural clay and enzyme masks. Test a patch of skin on your neck to make sure you can tolerate the mask without irritation. Ask for samples to try before you buy.

If I were stranded on a desert island, the two products that I would choose to have with me would be mascara and lip gloss. Burt's Bees makes wonderful lip balms and shimmers in a pencil form, and I love both Dr. Hauschka and Nvey Eco Organic Moisturizing mascaras.

tip 3:

Seek out mineral makeup. Hop on the bandwagon! Minerals are natural and do wonders for quickly adding a little glow. Mineral makeup protects your skin from the sun and environment.

They are available in foundation, blush, and eye shadows. Bare Escentuals, a leading manufacturer, offers a great selection of colors and textures to work with. You can also find Physician's Formula Organic Wear at your local drugstore. They make amazing bronzers and corrective concealers.

tip 4:

Don't forget your nails. Clear nail polish looks great on everyone. Nailtiques #2 is my favorite strengthener to keep nails long and strong with a little shine. You can also find natural nail polish and removers online or at your local health food store. Keep a luxurious cream on your nightstand and apply to hands and feet before bedtime.

tip 5:

Control blemishes. Treat that occasional blemish or skin irritation with the calming and soothing effects of a dab of lavender oil.

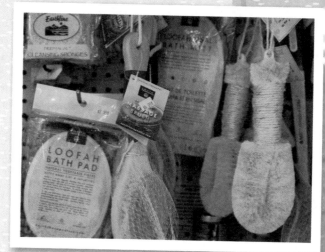

tip 6:

Keep your beauty tools clean. Wash makeup brushes and tools with baby shampoo every two weeks to avoid bacteria. P.S.: Organic baby shampoo is also the best makeup remover in the world.

tip 7:

Avoid beauty clutter. Use up every drop of your products before buying another one. You'll feel better about yourself. If something doesn't work for you, clear it out and give it away.

tip 8:

Water is the best beverage. The secret behind some of the freshest faces in show biz isn't what they put on, it's what they put in. Throughout your day, drink lots of water with lemon. Remember, water isn't Gatorade or "vitamin"-filled sugar drinks. Filtered water is your best weapon. When on the fly, choose Trinity, Smart water, or Penta water. Many other brands are nothing more than upscale tap.

tip 9:

Moisturize! Give your skin a drink, too. Regularly moisturize your body, face, hands, legs, and feet after drybrushing. Massaging with a light organic oil, lotion, or pure aloe vera gel is great for your circulation and keeps your skin soft and protected. My favorites include coconut oil, Fruit of the Earth Aloe Vera Gel, and pure shea butter from Whole Foods. All of these are available fragrance-free for sensitive skin types.

tip 10:

Catch Your ZZZZ's. Part of maintenance is knowing when to recharge. Everyone looks and feels better when they are rested and relaxed. Shoot for eight hours. Try and keep yourself on a schedule and respect it.

Guys can do this stuff, too. Don't worry, it doesn't mean you're gay. Or if you are gay, then you know the power of the tweezer!

All-Natural Makeup

Do you really know what's in the products you put on your skin? As much as possible, you want to use natural potions and lotions on your sexy epidermis. Many dangerous chemicals and toxins lurk in our beauty products. Being a detective starts with your diet, but it certainly doesn't end there. Remember, your body's largest organ is your skin. What you put on your body, you literally absorb. So if you wouldn't drink a bottle of Jergens, then don't put it on your body, because your skin will literally drink it in. A better choice—and one I use daily—is coconut oil. So luxurious!

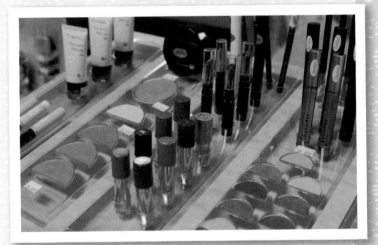

The average consumer babe uses dozens of personal care products per day! Many of those products contain hundreds of dangerous synthetic chemical compounds. Unlike (most of) the food and drugs we ingest, the cosmetics industry requires *no* pre-market safety tests, monitoring, or labeling. Due to massive loopholes in federal law, companies can put nearly any ingredient into your products. With statistics telling us that one-third of all men and half of all women will have cancer by 2050, it's important to investigate how exposures in our daily lives increase the risk of cancer.

Your makeup routine can expose you to more chemicals than your already taxed system can handle. I'm not saying you have to go naked—heck no! Instead, opt for natural products derived from plants and minerals. There are hundreds of selections out there to try. Here are a few of my favorites to get ya started:

- **PeaceKeeper:** Mineral lip paint, gloss, and polish!

- **Lavera Mascara:** No parabens, made using rose and jojoba. *Yum.*

- **Jurlique** makes great face moisturizer and other products, as does Dr. Hauschka.

- **Pangea Organics and Farmaesthetics** both offer luxurious body care and moisturizers!

- **Bee Yummy Skin Food** (live-live.com).

- **Care** by Stella McCartney.

- **No-Miss Nail Care's Almost Natural Polish Remover.**

- **Burt's Bees:** I love Burt's, especially the Replenishing Lip Balm with Pomegranate Oil.

- **Glominerals** (sold at Whole Foods). Great base and concealer.

- **Zia and Larénim** (that's *mineral* spelled backward) make great powders.

- **LUSH** handmade cosmetics, soaps, and bath care.

- **Essential Three** aromatherapy oils and products. Their merchandise is safe, luxurious, and downright yummy. Absolutely no synthetics used at all. Plus Caryn, the dynamic founder, is a cancer babe and I love her!

- **Young Living oils:** These aromatherapy products are among the best in the world. Their therapeutic grade oils are even good for internal use, as well as cooking, cleaning, first aid, and pet care.

One of the best places to browse natural cosmetics is Whole Body at Whole Foods. If there's one near you, try stuff on and play! Your skin, organs, and body will be glad you did.

Making a commitment to find the healthiest products for your body impacts more than just you. Natural products are better for the planet as well as your skin. Plus natural products aren't tested on our animal pals, either. Pooches, bunnies, and other loving critters will thank you! For more information, consult the Campaign for Safe Cosmetics, which works to protect and educate consumers on personal care products. Also, you can check the safety of the products you use by going to www.cosmeticdatabase.com.

skin art

Design your "I'm a courageous cancer biker" tattoo and pick a special place on your body to post it. Do you dare replace a breast with an angel? Why not? If you love your paint-free self, more power to you. But if cancer has made you feel disempowered and in need of a little pick-me-up, then find a nice motorcycle gang and ask the members for a few good recommendations. Remind yourself that you are a love warrior with heart and arrow. My dream tattoo is a butterfly; I know exactly where I want it, and one day I will have the guts to dig it into my skin. You are a canvas, your life is art, play! You don't have to go to the parlor. Thinking about inking can be fun enough. Go ahead, shake up the inner good girl.

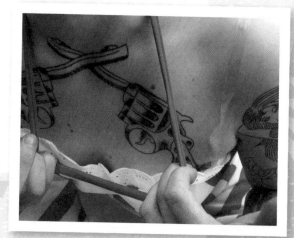

If you were stranded on a desert island, what two products would you choose to have with you? What are the ingredients in your favorite brands of these? Are there natural, organic, and/or mineral alternatives available? **Do the detective work!**

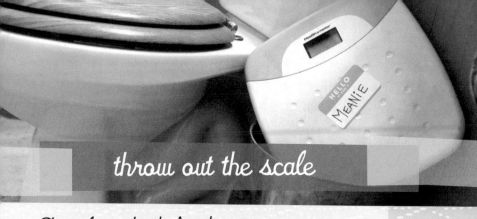

throw out the scale

The scale is a bunch of numbers that mean nothing and *everything*. That pesky, dangerous box is a booby trap full of good and bad news math. I hate math, I hate the scale. Back in the bun-head ballerina days I would measure myself constantly and then punish or praise accordingly. On punishment days I'd yack. Tis true, tis pathetic, tis my history; a golden nugget that makes me wise and human. However, that *box* is just that, a small container to cage ourselves. Prison is not sexy. No matter how it looks in the movies, prison is not a place to voluntarily visit.

Food: We adore it, despise it, worship and pray over it. We obsess and curse the voodoo grip it has over us. Food is the worst and best kind of lovah. Just when we think we've got it all figured out, stress and/or an emotional poop pie welcomes a malaise that lures us into a state of gluttony. When I used to eat meat I would speed through the drive-through dragging my scratched-up sage voice behind. "STOP! PLEASE! You're gonna regret it!" she'd shout. "Fuck off, you damn goody goody! I'm chowin'." Been there? Here's another one: At a recent CAT scan I got some terrific news. News I should have been very happy about. But since the scale barked numbers that I had never seen before, I couldn't help but spiral. How the heck did this happen? Where was I when those lbs hijacked my temple?

Let's focus less on our bodies and more on our perception of our bodies. Aren't we our harshest critics? Someone or something beat us up long ago. That moment has passed and yet we still carry the Louisville Slugger—and the scale.

For many of us, a healthy weight is not the one we're constantly chasing. It's the one we're at when we say, "Oh, if I could just lose five or ten pounds . . ." When I stop criticizing my numbers I have more free head-space to make and consume better meals.

Have you ever seen a picture of The Venus of Willendorf? Carved over 25,000 years ago, it's one of our earliest images of the human body. Lady Venus was found covered in red gunk on the banks Danube River, where she was likely made by some groovy locals during "me time" breaks from hunting and gathering. Back in the ice age, fat was in. Those folks appreciated junk in the trunk! A roomy pelvic girdle symbolized the future of the human race.

Extra pounds do not mean that you are a trainwreck. Some medications will stack you up like a human pancake. Do your best to feed yourself the optimum diet as discussed in this book and relax. If the problem is you're reed thin, there are many sound ways to return to a normal weight. More than likely you are experiencing a temporary symptom of your course of treatment. Grains, beans, nuts and nut butter, avocados, and coconut meat will add back some cushion.

Either toss the scale or use it as a signpost pointing you in the direction of knowledge and discovery. You know if you have a real problem that for health reasons must be addressed. The time to get serious is yesterday.

And while we're chucking stuff, throw out those stupid magazines that pollute our body image. They create what I

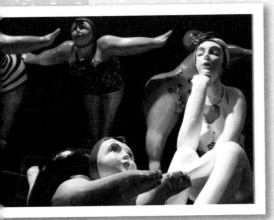

call the seesaw effect. One week we're too thin, the next, too fat. These magazines target and magnify the cellulite on unsuspecting vacationing celebrities. How dare she let down humanity! When we judge Miss Starlet we're measuring and judging ourselves. We're contributing to goddess oppression. Free her!

Hurricane Twinkie pig-out checklist

After much trial, error, and Scream Fests ('03, '04, '05, '06, the reunion tour of '07, and now '08), this is what I know for sure: Eating is a source of comfort and happiness for everyone! When life is out of control the easiest thing to grab is a snack. Snacks and feedbags = control. When babies realize that they have control over what goes in and out of their bodies, all hell breaks loose. Like everything else, it's a practice; it's a life long compassionate experiment. I can't sever myself from my problems, but I can work to get in front of them, to issue-spot and see them coming a mile away. The rains will pass, and when they do—get back on track. It's easy to see the neglect and "bad" choices. It's hard to see the good stuff, to pat ourselves on the back for our triumphs.

When the storm brews it's a sign that I am out of balance. Great revelation, but the damn storm is coming so what do you do? Prep yourself. Here's my state of emergency plan:

1. Junk OUT of my cabinets and fridge. I cannot be trusted.

2. Healthy snacks on hand, pre-cut/washed veggies and juice stuff prepped and ready in Tupperware containers.

3. Quick and easy side dishes ready and waiting to accessorize my big nightly salad. Rice pasta, quinoa, sweet potatoes, millet, soba noodles, garden burgers, hummus, Ezekiel bread, manna bread, etc.

4. Other staples, almond butter, tahini, nuts, oil cured olives and raw nuts, organic cold-pressed oils, hemp seeds, flax seeds, avocados, avocados, avocados . . .

5. Lots of yummy teas and lemon for my groovy lemonade, which I sip constantly (lemon, water, stevia).

6. Time carved out for smoothie/juice breaks.

7. A wee bit of fruit and healthy sweet treats (even though Dr. Ginger and all my other gurus say that canSer doesn't like sugar, I do, and I can't always say **no**).

8. A clean bathtub to hide in—with candles.

9. My rebounder out and ready for jumping.

10. A long walk ASAP.

How will you deal with the scale from this day forward? Make a plan and stick to it—not a diet plan, a how-to-deal-with-the-scale plan.

....

....

....

....

....

....

....

....

....

....

....

....

Going Steady (or a hot one nighter)

Should you date and if so how many dates should you go on before telling someone that you're a ~~patient~~ survivor?

This is a tough one, and there's no right or wrong answer. Here's what I know for sure: You ain't dead yet, sassy! Why put your romantic life on hold? Would going out and meeting someone of the opposite sex (even for just a chat) make you feel better? If so, then go. You may have to teach him or her that cancer isn't necessarily a death sentence and that no matter what fun you have smoochin' in the parking lot they won't catch it. Be patient, cancer makes us all realize that life isn't an endless party. However, this doesn't mean you allow yourself to be a doormat or to feel shame. HELL NO!

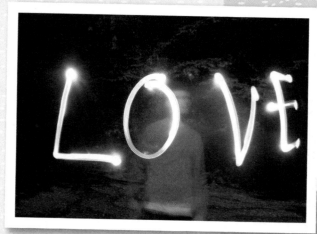

Timeless love stories are written when shared respect and adoration bring out the best in each of you. This love nurtures individual growth and builds a solid platform from which both parties can spread goodness in the world. Does the relationship make you better as a unit than you would be separately? If the answer is yes—fantastic! Go roll around!

If you're not ready to date, relax, take the pressure off. You'll have plenty o' time to sow your wild oats when you feel better. Again, trust the voice inside you. And if the person you're with doesn't have the backbone to stick it out during your darkest hour, then it's pink slip time. That's right, move on. Harsh but true. Genuine lovers don't drain our energy or create obstacles in our path. The wild ride ain't worth the costly repair job. This goes for friends as well. Life is short and cancer is hard. You do not have time for babies unless you are raising them. I know it's painful, but your recovery is crucial. Let nothing stand in your way.

One of my favorite wise women friends gave me solid advice after I got brutally dumped by a man who never saw my worth and didn't deserve my phenomenal Goddessness. "Girrrrl," she said with her Louisiana drawl, "bless him, thank him, and send that bastard to the light so you don't have to drag his tired ass around in your mind." Amen!

Is the man or woman you're with worthy of your awesomeness?
If you are single, what kind of partner do you wish to manifest in your life?
Put it out there, Cowgirl (and dude)—
ya gotta be in it to win it!

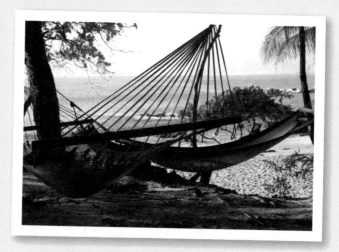

If you're not ready for some randy love, what are some things you need to feel confident enough to *open your heart?*

....

....

....

....

....

....

....

....

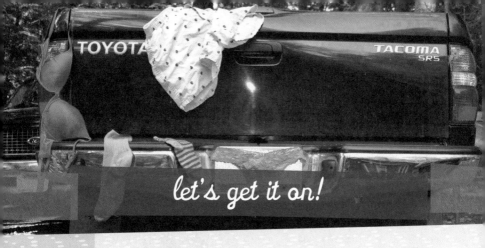

let's get it on!

Dating is one thing, getting naked is another! When I was first diagnosed, Kama Sutra was the last thing on my mind. My libido was in the deep freeze. Survivors often find that there is a big difference between dating post- and pre-cancer. When you're recovering from trauma, intimacy can make you feel raw and vulnerable. Plus, cancer treatments can cause embarrassing side effects. But there are lots of ways to get the engine started. Be creative: You have a new body now, so why not try something new to please it? Change the lens, flip the script; it's normal to feel like a mangled mess. Validate your thoughts by letting them out, but don't let them rule the roost! If you don't come to terms with how you've changed and who you are *now,* it will be harder to let someone else accept, love, and even touch you.

Cancer can ignite a sexual revolution if we let it. Burn your bra, baby (as long as it wasn't expensive). Why not get kinky? Stop blushing and buy some funky stuff. Lace, toys, and videos are around for a reason. When in doubt, repeat the following sentence: "I'm a supernova ass-kicking survivor, sexier than ever and ready to tango in the sheets." Hell yeah! Even if all you feel up to is lighting some candles and cuddling, turn it on. Don't sever a portion of your womanhood. Cancer helps us to go deeper, appreciate relationships more, and even create healthier role models for ourselves and our children. Open your mind to the possibilities of your life. Remember, you are not damaged goods, honey bunny;

you are a cancer *survivor* and thriver—physically, mentally, and spiritually!

Maybe some of you will recognize yourselves in Beth's story . . .

I didn't realize that I was the one shutting down the romance party. Quite simply, post-diagnosis I believed I was an unfit date. No man in his right mind would board a Love Boat cruise with me. Newsflash: They weren't rejecting me because of canSer, *I* was. Hang on, canSer does NOT equal Beth. Beth = funny, smart, kind, patient, sassy etc. Why *wouldn't* I put myself in the dating pool? CanSer hasn't made me "less than," it has strengthened me, empowered me, challenged me to grow. All those qualities make for one hell of a partner in my book.

Now what about sex? Initially I felt like my body was a virtual roadmap of scars. Who would want to navigate a highway with such bad scenery? How was I supposed to see my body as a palace of pleasure when I felt like it had double-crossed me? I knew I needed to redirect my focus away from the battle scars to the beauty that still remained. I deserved to swim in the endorphin/pheromone soup that romance creates. There's nothing better than when that dreamboat across the table is flirting with you. How invigorated, how alive does that make you feel? Now that's medicine! Dating, sex, and love are such integral parts of life, health, and vitality. Why in the world would I deny myself that? So here's my advice: Listen to Marvin Gaye singing "Sexual Healing" and obey that foxy man!

What does being *intimate* mean to you? Are you deciding whether or not you're worthy of loving and rubbing? Write 3 *beautiful things* about your body that any man or woman would be lucky to see and explore!

....

....

....

....

....

....

....

....

....

....

....

....

....

> **Strong women leave big hickies.**
>
> —MADONNA

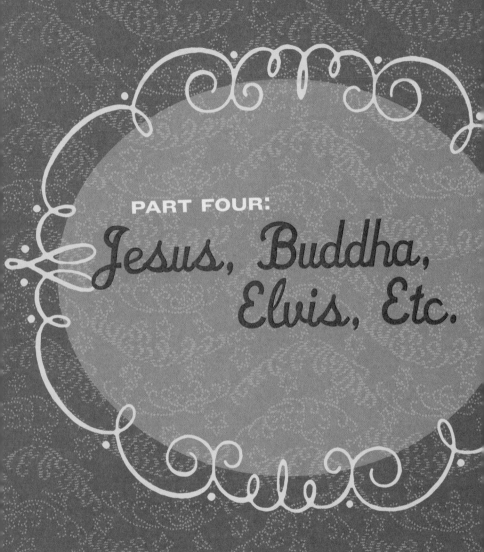

PART FOUR:

Jesus, Buddha,
Elvis, Etc.

What is prayer, how do I do it, when do I know if it's working, how long will this take me, and who the heck do I dial for a chat? Come on, I'm a modern woman and I want results!

When I first started thinking about "God," it felt very limiting. I was still confused, and the thought of saddling up to one dude/holy lady seemed like a mistake. What if God preferred to be called the Universe, Great Spirit, Goddess, the Light, or Herbie?

For years I let myself get so caught up in the correct salutation for the divine that I'd never get to the chatting. I would call the Big Whateva every name I could think of just in case. By the time I was done with the list, I barely remembered my prayer. After thirty-six years I finally surrendered to the word *God.* What a relief.

Does any of this sound familiar? What, how, and who you do it with are all irrelevant. The important thing is that you let yourself find the path that works best for you. Jump in, dabble, visit, read, write. Don't be a spiritual couch potato!

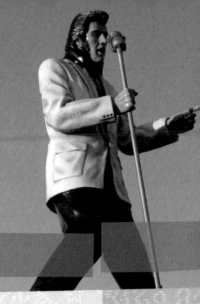

prayerpalooza!

Bring the fun back to prayer. Heck, as Justin Timberlake would say, bring the sexy back, too! Why does the process have to be so stiff and serious? Can you cartwheel your prayers, power-walk them? Can you slow-dance pray? Hacky Sack surrender? How about a chop and pray—every vegetable inspires a prayer. Amen. Plus, mindful eating and chewing makes the temple grub extra tasty and easier to digest. Grammar and etiquette are not essential for proper prayer, just be passionate.

Here's another golden goose egg: Balance asking with surrendering. Lay your burden down. Some common prayers in my queue look something like this:

God, please help me to walk in your light, to remember that I am a beautiful rose in the bouquet of your divinity, and that my mountainous problems are just temporary. Teach me compassion; remind me that my words and my speech contain great power, and to use them with good intention. Tap me on the shoulder when I make assumptions. Help me to love unconditionally and refrain from judging. I surrender my burden and lay it at your lotus feet, dear God. Thank you for taking it from me and composting it back to flowers.

The only real requirement for "successful" prayerpalooza is the willingness to open your heart and talk. Not an easy thing in this screwy era where showing our vulnerability is considered a weakness. But know this: There is no perfection in prayer. It is always available to us, and we don't get fewer spiritual Scooby Snacks by not doing it enough. When we pray, we tap into a huge chest of assistance. Ancestors and helpers lovingly remind us that we are part of a much bigger picture. Prayer casts a twinkling light to guide you through the dark times. Be willing to connect to something that is not predictable, something that holds the power to effectuate big and small shifts. Dare to scratch the surface and chat with the Great Whateva.

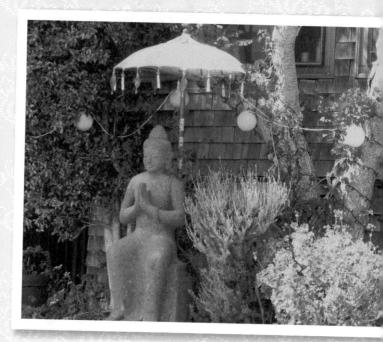

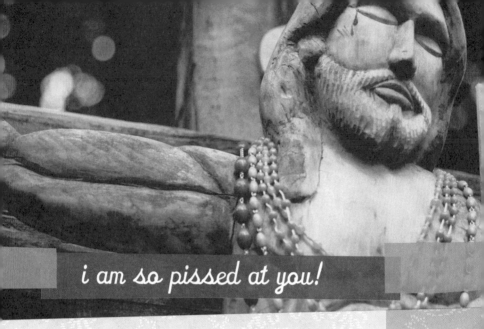

i am so pissed at you!

Perhaps you are peeved at God because of your diagnosis. We humans love to wag fingers, and it's frustrating when we can't pinpoint the blame. Where did this nightmare come from? Parents, genetics, cigs? Corporations, Dick Cheney, char-grilled beef? Hey, God, you suck! You were asleep at the wheel and you wrecked my life, ya big jerk. Guess what? It's okay to flip God the bird. Say nasty things and then duck. Just kidding! Nobody really has the answer to cancer (unless you were the Marlboro man) but it sure seems like someone is punishing us. Yet despite the pain, there is just too much beauty in the world. Personally, I don't think God is a nasty old crank sitting up in the sky trying to screw people.

CANCER IS HERE, SO NOW WHAT?

Now is the time to pick up the pieces and to move on. The grand ol' Whateva is there to teach us to believe in the God in everyone. *You* are the ultimate religion. Your family tree has divine roots. We come from the light and then spend a bunch of years living, learning, and stomping around in sneakers. Our job while in sneakers is to gather

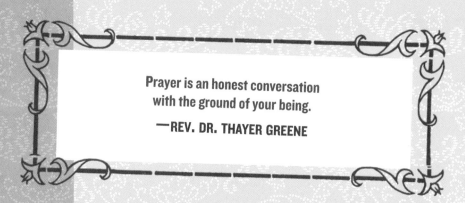

> Prayer is an honest conversation
> with the ground of your being.
>
> —**REV. DR. THAYER GREENE**

up as much knowledge and awareness as possible. One day we will all hear the holy chime signaling us that it's time to hitchhike back to the big mind, big heart.

People who croak for a minute and then write books about the experience all say the same thing: It is amazing over there! Well, if it's so frickin' amazing, then why do we come here in the first place? There must be a reason. It hurts over here, the prickers are bloody scratchy, and only masochists willingly sign up for pain.

What if the universe needs us? Perhaps we have a mission on Mama Earth. What if our very experience of suffering transformed into compassion and hate transformed into love has the power to raise the vibration of the universal? What if our time in sneakers adds an important ingredient to the divine chowder? If so, we return home bearing the energetic gifts of elevated consciousness and do-goodery. Our life force adds to the collective gigawatt. Boom!

Drop the Luggage,
EVEN IF IT'S GUCCI

Do you ever watch Animal Planet? Fascinating! Recently while spending my daily thirty-five on the treadmill, I watched as a mama baboon came to terms with the death of her only child. He was a spritely little chap with adorable Frisbee-size ears and a curiosity that kept Mama Monkey very occupied. Along came the leopard. Why does there always have to be a damn leopard?

All the baboons picked up their kids and scrammed up the trees. I knew where this segment was going because I work in television and the cuts and music cues were building to a throat-tightened crescendo. In the midst of the madness, the little chap fell to his death. Mama Monkey was so traumatized that she refused to believe her child had passed on. She carried her dead baby around for days, cleaning and preening, trying to will the little fella back to life. Finally on the third day the camera caught the stirring moment when Mama Monkey laid her burden down. After a last stroke, she said her goodbyes and scampered away.

As I marched on my treadmill, I was deeply moved by what I had witnessed. Sweat and tears poured down my face. I imagined my own mother, all mothers, and all children. I felt humbled and stung by my own instinct to move on. You can't go on mourning your loss forever, and sometimes your God can help you with the transition. I wonder whom the monkey prayed to?

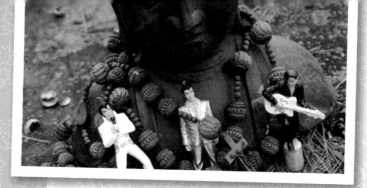

Yeah, Yeah, Sounds like a Bunch of Hooey to Me

Just because you're sick doesn't mean you need to find your savior. If prayer helps, start a conversation. If it doesn't, big whoop, make no judgments. Spirituality is a very personal trip. In my mind there is only one temple, one church, one mosque. We each go there in our own special way. It's an inner sanctum where you and your God high-five and catch up like old buds. Traditional religions don't resonate with everyone. There's a preconceived notion that when you are diagnosed, a lightbulb goes on and you suddenly realize what it's all about. You enjoy "the moment" more and live each day like it's your last. Well, that's a bunch of crap-o-la. First of all, I think it's better to live every day like it's your first . . . and it's so good that you can't wait for another. And furthermore, even though there is a golden cord that runs from me to my divine belief, I still scream at cabs and pout when my husband steals the remote in the middle of *Access Hollywood*.

WHAT SPEAKS TO YOU?
WHAT MAKES YOU FLOW?
WHAT GIVES YOU COMFORT?

You can find Jesus, Buddha, Elvis, etc, anywhere. Custom-design your spiritual trip. Remember, you alone have to do this work, but you don't have to do it alone. The trees can be your church. You can even find a spiritual practice in your relationships. A beach chair can be your holy ground or a cafe your ashram. It doesn't matter. The divine spirit is a wild pinto kicking inside you. Let her run.

What does **SPIRITUALITY** mean to you? Is there someone or something that gives you comfort?

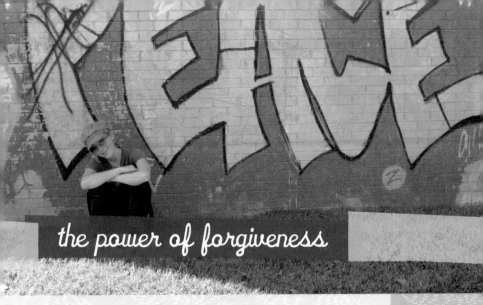

the power of forgiveness

Forgiveness is a central tenet in so many religions. But why do we still struggle with it? It sounds good from the Sunday pulpit but how many of us truly weave it into our lives? In Joan Borysenko's book *Minding the Body, Mending the Mind,* she says that "Forgiveness means accepting the core of all human beings as the same as yours and giving them the gift of not judging them." Borysenko teaches that forgiveness starts with ourselves and ripples out to others. Have you ever felt like you really hated someone? I have. For years I tried to forgive but I just couldn't. I felt tortured. So-and-so wronged me to the bone, and my only solution was to lash out in the twisted hope of making the evil-doer feel as bad as I did. But really the people you refuse to forgive hold you prisoner while they obliviously roam free. Here's the misperception: We see forgiveness as something we're doing for the other person, and since we're still darn hurt we don't want to give it up. This falsehood binds us to the pain. Let's get this clear, forgiveness is something we do for our own benefit first and foremost. This doesn't mean we have to invite them for dinner and make nice nice. Heck no! It means that we must pluck their talons from our hearts and let it go. Peace is a one-way ticket to wellness.

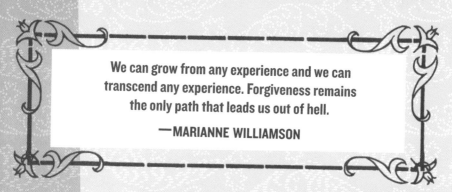

> We can grow from any experience and we can transcend any experience. Forgiveness remains the only path that leads us out of hell.
>
> —MARIANNE WILLIAMSON

Guess what's hardest to forgive? Your body. It betrayed you. After all you've done, this is the thanks you get? Hold on. Maybe it's time to appreciate the cancer? WTF?! Think about this, cancer isn't a terrorist with a bomb strapped to its back. Cancer is a response to a world spinning in the wrong direction. Can you love your tumors? Can you thank them? I see my beauty spots as little trashcans collecting debris so that the entire system doesn't shut down.

Here's another way to think about it: If cancer were a professor what would the lesson plan be? If you prefer to visualize exploding your cancer like it's a video game or melting a tumor like snow, go for it! There are so many ways we can connect out minds to our hearts in order to grow beyond our perceived limitations. The point is to become aware of the teaching and to then forgive your cells, your bones, your tissues—yourself.

Write a list of people and body parts you need to forgive. Write the lesson plan that cancer is teaching you. **CREATE** your own exercise that will allow you to let go and forgive. (You may need more paper for this.)

....

....

....

....

....

....

....

....

....

....

....

....

....

....

Dirt Naps

The terror of death is so powerful that most human beings will do anything to avoid even thinking about it. Unless we've flatlined, seen the light, and lived to tell the tale, most of us can only speculate about what the actual journey entails. For years the thought of death made me physically ill. A spooked out, jinxing paranoia grabbed my mind before it could wander into the void. At the time, I believed that worry was praying for what I didn't want, and since I didn't want to die, I refused to think about it. What if the worry could bring it on? Yikes, creepy, no thanks! Better to smoosh the heebie-jeebies than to play roulette.

However, anything that we hide grows in strength. If you refuse to allow yourself to taste extra-dark chocolate, the curiosity will one day get the best of you. Eventually, the temptation to explore the door in the floor became too great and I had to open my mind to the darkness. By allowing my imagination to drift and wonder, a very cool possibility floated to the surface of my frontal lobe. What if death is just like leaving a room? If you are willing to swim in this murky pond with me, read on; I promise the water isn't too deep and that I have a life vest and a first-aid kit in my bikini.

Picture this: You are at a party with your family and friends, and you are all really happy, eating crackers, and enjoying one another's company. You are laughing, hugging, and whooping it up. After a while you leave the room to go into another part of the house. Although you are no longer you with your friends and family physically, you can still hear them. Maybe you can even make out exactly what they are saying. No doubt Uncle Buddy is telling a great joke and Grandpa Harry is advising your sweet little sister to be careful.

You then open a different door to an area of the house even farther removed from the party. Now you can no longer hear your friends and family—but you know they are all still there, still in the house, still with you. Instead of hearing

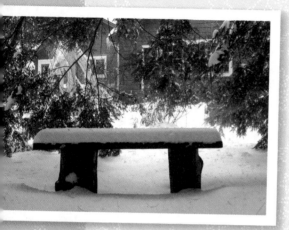

their laughter, you can now feel it. In fact, no matter where you go in the house, you feel their presence. You know that even though your physical relationship to them has changed, your energetic connection has not.

This last room is the universal God soup. The place where the saint tells us we're home; welcome to the new party. Jesus hands us butterfly wings, Buddha offers a bowl of rice and peas, and Elvis gyrates in white socks and sequins, offending no one.

Your what-if visualization will probably be very different from mine. Perhaps religion or a spiritual practice has given you a comforting model of what to expect when your last breath is exhaled. If you feel secure enough to explore this space, I encourage you to do so. I promise that worrying is not praying for what you don't want, and that the anxiety of the unknown can actually be more dangerous than a gentle fantasy.

I have no idea how the long dirt nap actually works, and to tell you the truth I don't want to find out anytime soon! But this visualization really helps me in rocky times of fear and doubt. Remember, death is the end of the chapter, not the end of the book.

> Death is not a period that ends the great sentence of life, but a comma that punctuates it to more lofty significance. Death is not a blind alley that leads the human race into a state of nothingness, but an open door which leads man into life eternal.
>
> **—REVEREND MARTIN LUTHER KING JR.**

WHAT HELPS YOU?

Can you picture death in a way that will give you peace rather than panic? If you could release your fear of death, what would your life look like?

....

....

....

....

....

....

....

....

....

....

....

....

....

....

....

....

....

....

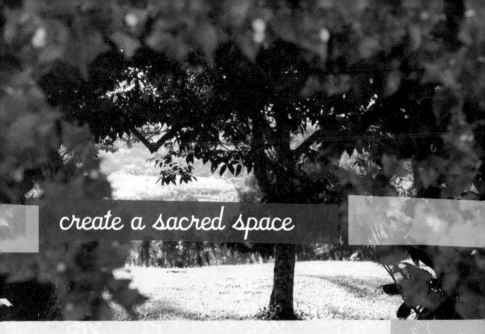

create a sacred space

Sacred spaces are like the chrysalis a caterpillar spins around herself for gestating. They are protective spaces where creativity and future plans bear fruit. The caterpillar dangles from a branch in her sacred space until she is ready to bust, move, and *fly, butterfly, fly.* You will, too.

It helps to have a corner of your home that feels sacred and is just for you. For the first year after my diagnosis, I spent about ten minutes every day in front of my little makeshift altar: just being there, feeling my butt on the pillow, taking deep breaths, and talking to myself. I was learning who I was, meeting my inner voice.

My mom has the grooviest altar. It is creative and mystical and always changes; like mini magic villages, each beckons you to explore. She has a gazillion gnomes, angels, feathers, rocks, talismans, and lordy knows what else. I do not snoop. The table is wired with big energy. Be respectful or *poof* you are a toad. Part mother, part priestess, the lady who birthed moi is a holy roller. As I thought about altars for this book, I knew I needed to go to the source of my education. If I left something out, I'd be in red-hot water. Take it away, Mom . . .

Big Kahuna Mama

A tall order to "take it away," missy! You're asking for a personal invitation to my inner sanctum where I have private secrets nobody knows about, not even you! But hey, for you, I would do just about anything . . . so here you go.

My altar makes me happy. It is my favorite thing in the whole world. If there were a fire in my home, I would single-handedly drag it out of harm's way, right after my husband and pets. It holds what is near and dear to me, the important, meaningful, and precious treasures that represent what I believe to be true and sacred in this world. I use it to voyage into my soul and find gold. I use it to prepare myself to receive the gifts of each day.

All the objects that grace my altar have been carefully chosen from my lifetime, and each one holds its own powerful energetic imprint. They inspire me, guide me, remind me of where I came from, and direct me to where I need to go to find happiness and fulfillment. Since it is my own creation, I can change it at any time. There are no mistakes on my altar, no judgments to hold me back. It is accessible and inviting. It comforts me and heals my wounds. It is my art and my refuge.

Daily visitations begin between 5:30 and 7:00 a.m. I start by lighting candles and burning incense. Then I settle down on my meditation cushion and write in my journal for about fifteen minutes. Next, I set an intention for the day and I decide what I will do just for me.

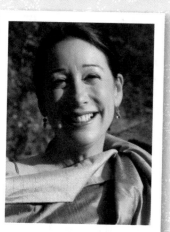

Following this ritual is meditation time. I ring my

little bell or sound a Tibetan singing bowl to bring myself into the present moment. Sometimes my husband joins me and takes charge of the bowl, but most times I am alone. Occasionally I cast the I Ching or Celtic Runes to entice my unconscious to send up some good advice. My meditation lasts about fifteen minutes and ranges from excruciatingly difficult to gloriously quick and easy—and I have no way of tracking how it will go. I trust that it has unseen, unquantifiable pluses, so I just keep doing it.

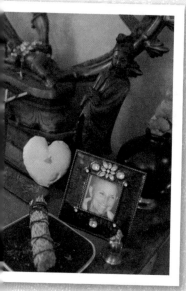

My altar

I love this time of day. Nothing important has to happen. I can just press PAUSE on the outside world and connect to the invisible realm where lots of wonderful things are waiting to blossom. Somehow the veil between the worlds slowly lifts to allow space for my own imagination to be present. Nothing is ridiculous or outrageous; everything is enough, nothing is too much.

Sometimes I neglect my altar, as I do myself. Sometimes I court it with beautiful fresh flowers and new aromatic candles. Some days are cleaning days, when I dust and move things around to get the energy flowing again. Other times, when I am feeling blue, I just sit there and look at the sacred objects and ask them to work their magic. On any given day, they have the power to rekindle warm and cozy feelings confirming, without a doubt, that I am loved, valued, and appreciated. At any given time, there are serious and funny cards on my altar that carry loving words and sentiments,

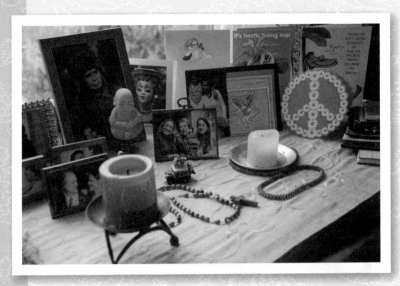

Mom's altar

reminding me that I am here for many reasons and have special work to do.

On my altar there are photographs of those near and dear to me. Some of my ancestors who have passed are mixed in with my beautiful daughters, my loving husband, and my top informants, Thich Nhat Hanh and Padre Pio. They all remind me that I am part of a long lineage, a much bigger picture. There are also a couple of pictures of me on display. One from when I was eight years old, to remind me to keep the child within me alive and well, and another picture of myself from my most glamorous years, to keep me on my toes!

Statues of the big guns, C, B, and G (Christ, Buddha, and Ganesh), along with angels and fairies, also grace my altar at different times. There is a silver mirror, which I use to periodically take a close look at myself (and I don't mean the wrinkles here). I have a Shiva Lingham stone from the sacred Narmada River, one of India's seven holy sites. Kristin giggles and says it's a phallic symbol, but to me it is a beautiful stone that traveled

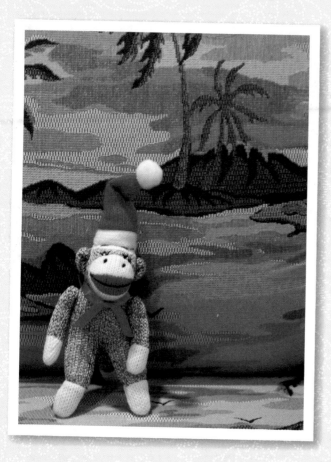

from the other side of the world to rest on my
altar. I have holy water from the Sanctuario de
Chimayo in New Mexico and my very special sock
monkey witch, Lorenza, and bobbing Buddha (really meant for the dashboard of a car); both make
me laugh out loud and not take life too seriously.

And then there are my most treasured posses-
sions, the ones that sit in my power bowl, lovingly
handcrafted by a childhood friend, Carmen. A gold
locket engraved with my nickname, given to me
by my mother the Christmas before she died. In it
live her picture and the thin gold wedding band
that she wore for fifty years. A little silver tooth

fairy bell that holds just a pinch of her ashes, a powerful reminder that death is the other side of life. A lighter imprinted with the name of my father-in-law's company, uncovered by my husband at a flea market a couple of weeks after his dad's death, surely a final gift that was sent with a father's love.

And then there is my most cherished possession of all, a "diamond" ring given to me by Kristin when she was seven years old. She had saved five dollars that year to buy me this extravagance for Christmas. I can clearly remember the excitement that only a child can show trying so hard to keep such a surprise a secret. It is priceless to me, forever holding the powerful energy of my daughter's love. Lastly, over the bowl rests a single feather, meticulously carved from a moose antler by a Sioux Indian I never met, but whose strength has graced my life through his beautiful art. I placed the feather on my mother's abdomen as she passed on to her next great adventure. For me it holds the imprint of her last breath.

Lots of stories, lots of feelings and connections, all spread before me on my altar in the stillness of morning time. Each sacred object carries its own unique and precious energy. Combined they hold the memories that are the fabric of my life. My altar lives and breathes. It expands and contracts. Sometimes I am receiving and sometimes I am giving. At my altar my heart opens and comes to rest in peace. It is my table—where I go to receive nourishment, to celebrate, to mourn, to be with myself. It teaches me to be mindful, to pause and wait with confidence for the answers will come in their own time. I remember my strengths at my altar and when I come to a crossroad, I pray for guidance.

My wish for you is that you give yourself the powerful gift of your own altar and wait patiently for the epiphanies to come. They always do.

Altar Power

Your altar can be as humble or as grand as you wish
to make it. It is a personal creation, a work of art.
Let it be a reflection of you. Large or small, it will
be a place that you have designed to hold power for
yourself. Just start building it, one meaningful object
at a time. Then let your precious treasures simmer
together and become even more powerful and sacred
as you honor them. Here are a few thoughts and suggestions to get you started:

- **Altar.** My altars have been many things
over the years—shelves, windowsills,
breakfast trays, stools, benches . . . use
your imagination. If you spend a lot of time
in your car, altar your dashboard. If you
travel a lot, make it compact and portable.
Currently my altar is an antique Chinese
sofa converted to a coffee table.

- **Altar cloth.** Your altar can be left simply
as it is or covered with a special fabric,
perhaps a doily made by your grandmother's hands. I have draped my mother's silk
embroidered shawl over mine. You can use
place mats or table runners. I like to use
something that is handmade and holds
ancestral energy.

- **Power bowl.** You might want a special
bowl to hold the most precious treasures on
your altar.

- **Photographs of ancestors,** family, deities,
and gurus add inspiration and support to
your altar.

- **Cards received** from special people in your
life act as reminders of how special you are.

- **Statues of your favorite deities**, saints, angels, fairies, power animals—whoever or whatever resonates for you, let them grace your altar. They will come when you call them. On my altar I have a small wooden Buddha, a white porcelain angel that belonged to my mother-in-law, a little ceramic skunk, and a white swan (two of my power animals).

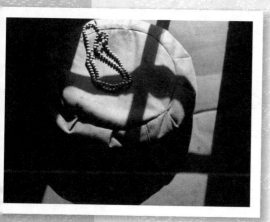

- **Incense or sage.**
- **Candles.**
- **Crystals.**
- **A bell or Tibetan singing bowl** to signal the beginning and end of your meditation.
- **Beads** of any kind. They can be rosary beads or perhaps sandalwood prayer beads.

- **Offerings** in the form of flowers, or anything collected from nature such as stones, shells, or beautiful leaves.

- **A meditation cushion** or pillow to sit on.

- **A shawl** handy to keep you warm (the one I use belonged to my mother).

- **A storage place** for the precious things you may want to rotate. To one side of my altar, I place a little chest with different-size drawers to hold the many cards and special things I use to grace my space.

- **A clock** so you know how long all this is taking!

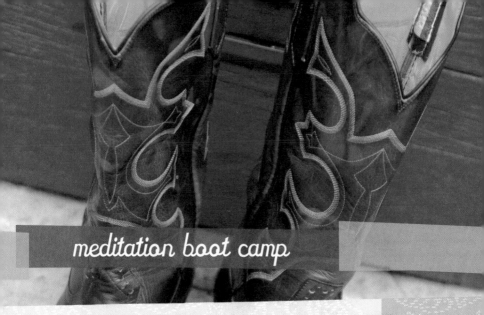

meditation boot camp

If you've ever taken a yoga class, you've experienced those annoying five minutes at the end when you're forced to inhale "let" and exhale "go." For me those last minutes were always torture. Me meditate? If I sat still, I'd snap!

Pilgrimages to zendos, ashrams, sweat lodges, churches, and retreats can really help the inward zoo. The silence within those walls reminds us that beneath our static lies an encyclopedia of healing guidance. Calm . . . Can you picture it? What a nice place to take a day trip! It's free, our organs get a rest, and the view is spectacular.

The thought of meditating sometimes overwhelms people. Some fear it will bore them to pieces and take forever. Others are afraid of what they might see and hear if they took the time to pay attention. It's not rocket science. You probably won't have a Cecil B. DeMille–style spiritual awakening à la Moses in *The Ten Commandments*. The benefits of meditation are much subtler than that, yet they hold similar grandeur. You can space your time outs—or should I say "time ins"?—throughout the day. You can even meditate while you pee. Why not? What else do you have to do? Sit, pee, take a deep breath, and empty your mind.

Meditation first guides our focus to our breath and then to our higher purpose. The space between the chatter is where your healer lives. Quiet the din and introduce yourself. *Hi me, I'm me. Nice to meet you!*

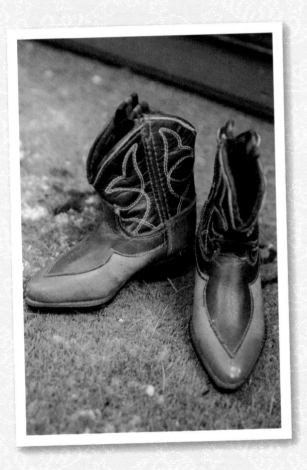

The Busy Person's Guide to Stopping

So you've decided to go inside and wrangle the monkey mind rodeo, huh? Good luck! Before you jump in, here are a few suggestions that may prevent madness.

Buy a kitchen timer or a meditation chime. Go to your sacred space. Find a comfortable seat on a pillow or chair. Set the timer for an appropriate number of minutes to start with, let's say five to ten. Close your eyes and begin to count to ten. The inhale is one—then exhale one; inhale two, exhale two; and so on. If your mind drifts and you find yourself buying shoes or guns, gently bring it back and start counting again. Your mind is like a muscle: The more consistent you are, the better your results. String the time and the days together like pearls on a necklace.

Each time you return to the breath, you break an old pattern (distraction) and create a new mental habit (focus). Direct your mind where you want it to travel instead of always going for the ride. You can also use the mantra if that is easier for you. For example, inhale "let" exhale "go." Or inhale "may all beings everywhere," exhale "be happy and free." If you know Sanskrit, then by all means do it old school. *Om namah shivaya!* In Zen Buddhism the power of concentration is called Joriki. Joriki starts on the inside and radiates out to all aspects of your life. But in order to experience the strength and power it creates, you must practice on a regular basis.

How many of you are holding your breath right now? Do a body scan. Now exhale. When we are stressed, the first thing we do is tighten, gasp, and shut down. Most of us don't realize that we're walking around in a constant state of tension. We equate our high levels of stress with normalcy. Unless you grew up under a lotus tree, your adrenal glands look like Keith Richards on a bad day. Breathe now. Narrow your focus to what really matters: *you!*

Believe it or not, there is a right and a wrong way to breathe. Rapid, shallow breathing—the way most people suck in oxygen—can lead to a host of health problems, both physical and mental. Learning to breathe properly ensures that your body is getting all the delicious oxygen it needs. When you're breathing properly, your stomach, not your chest, rises slightly as you breathe in. When you exhale, your stomach lowers slightly. *Note:* Poor posture restricts the flow of air and the rise and fall of your diaphragm. So remember your mother's nagging and sit up straight!

How's your breathing?
How's your posture?

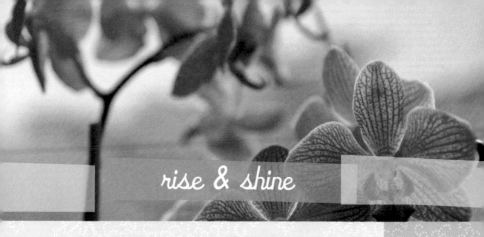

rise & shine

Let me throw out a few potential plot lines for starting your day. Which one sounds most appealing?

scenario one:

You rocket out of bed late, pour a pot of coffee down your throat, and race to your computer. Your mind downloads pages of the horror, politics, celebrity cellulite, and rising interest rates, while your pits start to sweat from caffeine blowout. Oh my God you haven't checked your e-mail yet! Like a Xerox machine, you quickly scan the notes from cyberwhiners who remind you of all the things you failed to accomplish yesterday.

Then you nearly break your neck as you swan-dive into the shower for a lightning-fast hose-off, and race to work (without breakfast). If you have a gaggle of kids, double the chaos factor. If you have a dog, triple it. If you have a cat and a husband, you're screwed. You never feel rested, you have no idea how to connect with your inner wisdom, and the damn days are never long enough. A warm tub and a few seconds of peace feel like a one-way trip to the Bahamas.

scenario two:

Because you went to bed at a reasonable time and clocked eight full hours of restorative sleep, you wake up at 5:30 or 6:00 a.m. feeling happy and

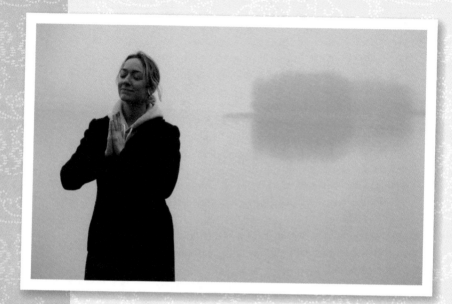

refreshed. You then pour yourself a cup of herbal tea, look out your window to see if the bunny who lives in your garden is dining on your weeds, and head over to your sacred space. Once you are comfortably seated and the sage is blazing, you turn to some uplifting spiritual material to fill your reservoir. Perhaps you tickle your gratitude journal with some thank-yous, amens, and affirmations. You close your eyes and meditate for ten to thirty minutes. As you come to your senses and your center, you realize that there is no need to rush. You have more than enough time to get your work done, and nothing will rattle you. You then bounce off to the bath and emerge renewed and ready for the conscious inhales and exhales that will fill the next twenty-four hours.

scenario three:

Invite yourself to find the middle ground. We are all stumbling around doing the best we can. We can't get rid of all the deadlines, but we don't have to murder ourselves to get the job done. Perseverence.

Consistency. Small steps. Make choices that honor your needs first and foremost. Carve out what is most important to you and protect it like a lioness. Remember, you are the CEO of your life. If you limp to the finish line with your pancreas dragging behind on the asphalt, what was the point? Living in the now allows us to experience each and every one of our seconds. Time ticks by for everyone, not just for those with cancer. While you're driving, rinsing your hair in the shower, switching the wash into the dryer, breathe it in and notice your magnificent life. Hallelujah! Pass the spiritual pancakes.

Your beautiful mind is the most open in the morning, which is why it's helpful to start your day with centering exercises such as meditation.

What three changes can you make in your morning routine?
Describe them. Which is most important?

Pillow Power

To truly let go of something, we must see it first. Quieting your mind and turning your attention inward leaves you naked with yourself. As the masterfully suppressed head junk reveals itself, you may feel a frightening sense of exposure. Ooh la la! Drop your skivvies and allow yourself to sunbathe in your Zen birthday suit! Let the rays fall on the pale places that have been swaddled in jeans and long underwear. When you're ready to cover up again, wrap yourself in a gorgeous fabric of your choosing. Scattered minds pick polyester; centered minds choose organic cotton. The gutsy folks who sit their ass on the pillow will tell you that the junk that does not serve you will present itself with a deep moan. If this happens to you, don't freak out. Moaning is good; fun at times.

As you begin to peel the layer of your onion, there may be some tears and tantrums. Fantastic! Allergic reactions to focus and concentration are normal. Once you practice with regularity, you will find Wonder Woman strength in your ability to gather your attention. A lasso and an invisible plane await you as you transform from road rage bitch to an enlightened navigator, unshaken by the parade of jackasses who constantly cut you off.

THE ONLY AGREEMENT THAT YOU MAKE WITH YOURSELF IS TO LET GO OF ANY JUDGMENT YOU MIGHT HAVE ABOUT HOW WELL YOU ARE ACCOMPLISHING THIS NOT-SO-SIMPLE TASK.

Your mind will wander, and when it does, do not grab your mental whip and begin to chase your thoughts with the intention of catching them for a beating. Instead, cozy up and settle in. What works for me may not work for you. There is a wide range of bite-size pauses that will add space to your life. Try mindfully folding your laundry or doing the dishes. Stop for one minute and stand still in the sun. Tap into the sound of the water while sitting in front of a trickling fountain. You don't have to be a monk in a cave to add a little Zen-fabulous to your life.

As you further your practice, you may awaken to the cosmic glue that holds us all together. The word *yoga* means union or "to yoke"—as in, with the divine. Wow, yoking with the divine, when was the last time you did that? Kinky! Don't be surprised if a string of Christmas lights flicker on in your newly conscious mind. When I dove in, my connection to the world around me grew so strong that it became too painful to turn my back; to do so would be to abandon myself. The choices I make have an impact on my inner and

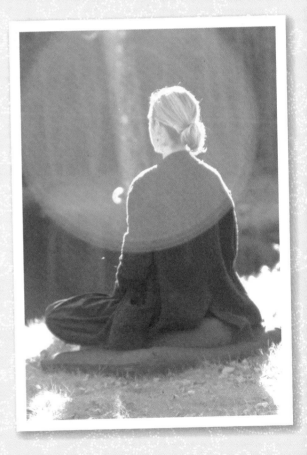

outer environment. Global warming doesn't just take place in theory, out there, on Al Gore's video projector. It happens right under your skin in the unbalanced and deforested terrain of your body. Now, that's food for thought! Basically, separation of any kind stinks!

WHAT'S THE OLD ZEN HOT DOG JOKE?

Make me one with everything.

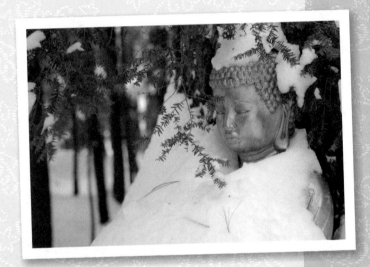

Meditation is not relaxation spelled differently.
—JON KABAT-ZINN

HOMEWORK ASSIGNMENT:

Meditate. Just do it! What was it like? Where did your mind drift to? How did you bring it back?

....

....

....

....

....

....

....

....

....

....

....

....

....

....

....

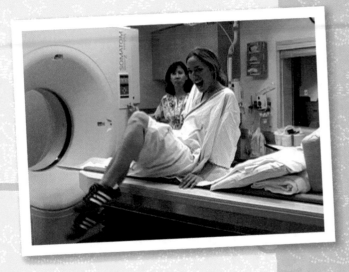

scan day

No matter how centered you get, scan day will wring you like a spin cycle. Try meditating on the CAT scan bed. I have a tribe of protectors on the other side, and they all come wearing white, banging drums, smokin' peace pipes (filled with *good* green grass, and not the wheatgrass kind), and creating sacredness. When Team Spirit arrives, no matter what happens I am not alone.

Thoughts from My Lil' Sis

When my clan read a draft of my spirituality section, it ignited a great debate and some juicy conversation. Olé! Cha, cha, cha, I love that! Leslie (my sister in shrink school) offered some righteous vocal cord slapping to add to our philosophical family chew-over. Check it out.

Meditation for me comes in moments, preferably short in duration, and often when there is nothing else to do. I like to meditate most when I'm walking or when I'm by myself commuting somewhere. Take a train, for example. When I'm on a New York City subway train and I'm pissed because I can't sit down, my bag is heavy, and the angry man next to me won't shut the hell up, I close my eyes. Rather than fighting against it, thinking over and over about how much I wish my stop would come, I actually do the reverse—I embrace the moment in all its shitty glory. I am right here, right now. I listen to the man complain, and to the sounds of the train as it rocks back and forth underneath me. I focus on my breath and feel my body as it exists—my clothes brushing against me,

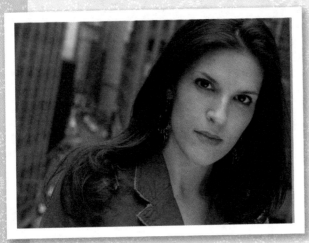

maybe even hugging me in places that I wish they didn't. I am present. For better or worse, this is where I am.

We spend so much time living in our thoughts rather than our reality. When we're driving to the grocery store, we're thinking about what we're going to make for dinner. While we're making dinner, we're thinking about what we're going to do after that. I try to remind myself to not just listen, but hear; to not just look, but see; to not just breathe, but live. Whatever is happening in this moment, it's the only time it will ever be.

That's some good stuff! Of course I taught Leslie everything she knows and take full credit for her cool factor. I wish! Your family has more wisdom than you think. Tap the tree.

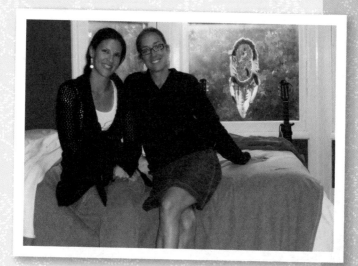

What's your favorite meditation place?
What's the lousiest? How can you be mindful in each?

....

....

....

....

....

....

....

....

....

....

....

....

....

....

My soul sister Sera and I were separated at birth. We are still scratching our heads and trying to figure out how our parents kept this information from us all these years. The 1970s were a wild time, but come on! Sera is a red goddess and word chef who creates tasty recipes of spiritual freedom for the modern woman. A Harvard-trained scholar of mysticism and comparative religion and an intrepid spiritual cowgirl, Sera wrote *The Red Book: A Deliciously Unorthodox Approach to Igniting Your Divine Spark*. Put it on your Crazy Sexy Syllabus, folks. It's a must-read for jailbreaks and sacred galloping. Yeehaw! Here's Sera's take on meditating . . .

Spiritual Mad Libs, by Sera J. Beak

A playful game of what I call "Spiritual Mad Libs" is best practiced as a meditation afterglow—after you've completed some sort of practice that relaxes your body and mind, and puts you in a quiet and centered space. The energetic focus of this exercise is listening to your red-hot heart, the cozy home of your authentic self, your divine spark, your inner healer—the Grand Central Station for Your Powers That Be. When you take the time to calm your mind and let your awareness slip down into this conscious heart realm, you'll find that it has quite a lot to say—or rather, *you* have quite a lot to say to yourself. You can connect with your heart simply by placing your hand on your chest for a few moments, closing your eyes, and feeling your heart beat.

A few important tips:

- Throughout this exercise, if you don't sense or hear a freakin' thing, I want you to *make it up*—pretend you are connecting with your heart and hearing insightful information from your inner healer. (Try imagining that you have a wise and loving authentic self, and she's gabbing intimately with you over coffee. What would she share with you?) This pretending isn't fake or false; it helps to create a pathway for your experience—using your imagination is often the first step in igniting or tapping into any new spiritual awareness.

- Your authentic self doesn't boss you around or have a weak, angry, bitchy, spiteful, or negative tone (that would be the voice of your ego, or your fears). Your authentic self is a wise and loving aspect of you. Although she maybe a wise*ass* at times and even sport a dirty sense of humor, her words should always be accompanied by a warm, powerful, and unconditionally loving energy.

- Don't overanalyze the sentences that follow. Don't overthink your answers—let your heart speak uncensored, even if the answers initially seem silly or strange. Let your self flow.

When you're ready, grab a pen, take a deep breath into your heart . . . and let's roll. Pretend your inner healer—however you imagine her to be—is speaking these sentences to you while encouraging you to draw from her well of compassion and wisdom to finish them.

My love for you is like . . .

....

....

....

....

....

....

....

....

If you would just remember that . . .

....

....

....

....

....

....

....

....

I feel **the most connected** to you when . . .

....

....

....

....

....

....

....

....

I feel disconnected **from you when . . .**

....

....

....

....

....

....

....

....

....

....

What can you do each day to help build and strengthen your relationship with me? A simple meditation practice? A walk in nature sans iPod? **Dancing in the living room? Gardening? Journaling?**

....

....

....

....

....

....

....

....

....

....

....

....

....

....

....

....

Every time you see or hear
THIS WORD OR PHRASE
(on a sign, a song, online, on TV, wherever),
know that it's a little divine wink from me, a
thumbs-up from your inner universe, a little
love pat on your spiritual booty.

Right now, the most important thing
you need to know about **your life** is . . .

These particular open-ended statements are meant to help you reestablish a more fluid connection to your authentic self, but once you're comfortable with this form of communication, you should create your own spiritual Mad Libs—from broad open-ended sentences to more precise fill-in-the-blank questions. They can be as funny or serious, shallow or deep, broad or specific as you want, and they can be about anything—from health advice to food choices to relationships to sex toys—no subject is taboo or off limits. Just try to make sure you're relaxed and centered when you fire away. Bottom line: Your inner healer is always dishing, constantly communicating with you; all you gotta do is tune in and let 'er rip.

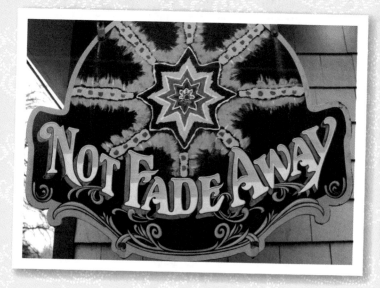

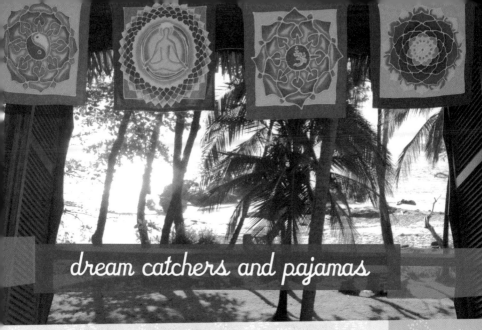

dream catchers and pajamas

Dreams are mysterious gifts wrapped in hidden meaning. As you remove the nightly paper, you release the offerings from your unconscious. Dreams are soul stars revealing a map of inner constellations and direction. *Should I go right? Do I go straight? Did I make a wrong turn back at the 7-Eleven?* Your dreams will tell you.

The year before I was diagnosed, I had a *master dream*. Those are the dreams that guide and shape your life. That dream of mine is the reason I'm writing this book today. I was with a group of photographers on an excursion into the wild. We walked for what seemed like days until we finally approached a dark tunnel. There were two choices: Go into the unknown or take the longer path around it. Though everyone advised against it, I picked up my camera, brought it to my face for protection, and walked straight into the darkness. As I did thousands of monarch butterflies flew past me, gently caressing my face with their delicate (and thunderous) wings. The farther I walked, the more butterflies appeared, until finally they guided me to the sun-kissed light of a beautiful green meadow.

Monarch butterflies are symbols of freedom, joy, and creativity. Their brilliant orange color reminds me of shape-shifting monks' robes flapping about, ready for resurrection. These beautiful winged creatures travel vast distances (up to 3,000 miles round-trip), flying in large groups to return home, often to the very same tree. Native American legends say that if you have a secret wish, find a butterfly and whisper your wish to it. When you release the butterfly, it will carry your wish to the Great Spirit. By setting the butterfly free, you are helping to restore the balance of nature, and your wish will surely be granted.

Orange is the color of the second chakra, which connects to sex, power, and rock and roll. It relates to your ability to connect to the being inside and to hear what your body wants and needs. When I got the cancer news, I remembered my dream and immediately saw it as a sign to document my journey. The butterflies were telling me something. I named my dream *Psychic Wings* and realized that it was a signal from the deepest corner of my toes. Naming your dreams helps to stimulate the juice.

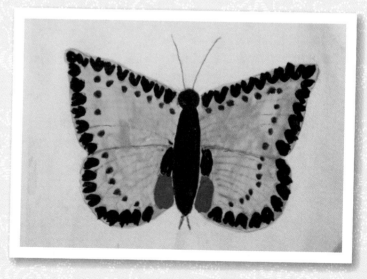

If your dreams were BUMPER STICKERS, what would they say?

....

....

....

....

....

....

....

....

....

....

....

....

You see things; and you say, "Why?"
But I dream things that never were; and I say, "Why not?"

—GEORGE BERNARD SHAW

Sera has some great sister vision about the power of dreams; here's a little ditty for your next zonk trip.

Dreams
by Sera J. Beak

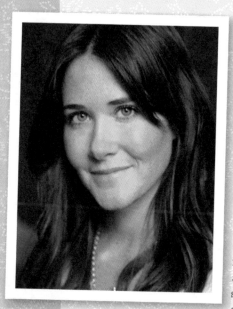

Last night, when you were snoozing and the stars were twinkling, the universe was conspiring in your favor. 'Tis true. When you shut your eyes and the world fell away and you wandered off into dreamland, this is exactly when the universe began to offer you invaluable guidance by speaking to you in the richest language she knows: signs, symbols, metaphors and feelings, telling images and fertile scraps of memory. Why is your inner universe putting on such a rich and colorful nightly show? Because she knows that dreams, if properly explored and heeded, can help transform you into the superheroine you were born to be.

Many believe that dreams are revelatory mirrors, reflecting your mental, emotional, spiritual, and physical health in ways no CAT scan or blood test ever will. (Personally, I often think of dreams as alternative health plans that aren't covered by mainstream medical modalities.) When you fall asleep, your conscious mind loosens its grip, allowing your unconscious—the part of yourself you're not directly aware of, but are indirectly influenced by—to come forward and show you what's *really* up with your life, steering you toward aspects of your relationships, career, sexuality, spirit, family, and physical health that might need a little (or a lotta) TLC.

Our light and our dark, our hopes and our fears (hello, nightmares), our beauty and our ugliness all show up in our dreams. They're a bit like cryptic, mystical CliffsNotes on how to become whole, and the great thing is, if we take the time to study the content of our dreams, we can better come to know who we really are, and even start making clearer, healthier, more conscious choices about how we want to live. Dream work (and play) invites body, mind, and spirit to engage in an energized threesome, which in turn can make our innate healing powers that much more available to us.

Whaaa?

"Yeah right," you might reply. "What's so insightful about the whack dream I had last week, in which I was naked and dragging around a bunch of heavy plastic bags as I wandered aimlessly around some weird McMansion while annoying animated penguins kept waddling by my feet? Mystical healing revelations, my ass."

I hear you. But first off, never dismiss or underestimate your dreams, no matter how silly or Alice-in-Wonderland surreal they may initially appear. Second, taking your dreams literally is a bit like taking an old Bible story literally—rarely a good idea, as there's almost always more simmering beneath the allegorical surface. That's why, when it comes to interpreting our dreams, we need to become astute metaphorologists (kin to meteorologist, but with better outfits).

Let's take the above dream as our example: Being naked in a dream often means feeling open, unprotected, vulnerable, free of excess guises, or perhaps emotionally bare or raw. A house or building you're wandering in could reflect the enclosed space of your mind, soul, heart, or body, whereas individual rooms might reflect new places inside yourself to discover and explore. See if you can note the details. What's their size and shape? How are they decorated: Empty or cluttered? Shabby chic or Zen? Are there any doors or windows? Are they open or closed tight?

As for those garbage bags, those could reflect excess baggage that your inner healer (aka your inner universe, which winks from your unconscious) is alerting you about—perhaps frightening medical statistics, financial worries, your family's concerns, old emotional wounds, all sorts of lingering weight you drag around without really knowing it. (Because dreams come from our unconscious, they're excellent at giving insights we might not be so open to receiving in our waking life.) And as legit as some of that weight may be, it could be sucking too much of your vital energy and slowing down your healing process.

And the penguins? Well, who knows what their symbolic significance is, but if you dreamed about them, your psyche sure as hell has some idea (see below for tips on how to interpret your funky dream imagery). Of course, they could just be the remnants of that rerun of *Happy Feet* you saw on HBO last night, maybe reminding you that it's okay to lighten up now and then, no matter how much ice you gotta traverse in life.

Bottom line: Transform your dream images into metaphors for your life. Allow these images to marinate in your intuitive juices. Take the time to learn the language of your soul. Become fluent in symbolese. You never know what you might learn.

Dream Magic

One slightly controversial, but important thing to mention here: It's not uncommon for some people to link their physical healing directly to a particular dream. I've read numerous accounts of dreamers hearing very specific information, such as someone's name or a random keyword they've never noted before, in their dreams, which led them to a special doctor or inspiring book or even a new medicine that radically helped their healing process. I've even heard stories in which a mythological character or past relative made an in-dream appearance and "touched" the dreamer on a part of the body that needed to be examined in waking life. Truly, the dream state can be a very powerful realm.

Let me be clear: I don't relay these examples to impress you or make you feel like crap because you think your dreams aren't up to par, or even to make you worry that your inner healer is broken or MIA, off slurping piña coladas in Cabo while you're tossing and turning and dealing with "real" life. Rest assured, no matter what you're dreaming, no matter how undramatic or forgettable you think your dreams may be, the potential for healing is always present. I share the above examples because I think it's important to keep ourselves primed and open to the idea that our body, mind, and spirit look for *all sorts* of ways to help us heal. Our inner healer doesn't always play by medical rules, statistics, or theories.

One thing to keep in mind: Your unconscious takes direction very well. You can set an intention to receive more healing juju from the dream world. Try this: Before you fall asleep, simply make a heartfelt request to your inner healer (say it aloud, whisper it, write it down, whatever works for you): *I'd like to experience healing tonight,* or *Show me some clear information about reclaiming my health,* or some other phrase that resonates with you, like *Bring it!*

Once you start showing your inner healer that you're taking her seriously and you're bringing more kindling in your dream world, she will most definitely bring the fire, but you need to trust what does or does not show up. Remember, your individual process of healing is as unique as your fingerprint. What works for others very well might not work at all for you, and vice versa. But no matter what, healing (not necessarily *curing*) happens quite naturally when we take steps toward knowing (and being) who we truly are. Paying close attention to dreams is a powerful step in that direction.

Dreaming through the Ages

If any of this sounds a little new agey woo-woo, know this: Healing by way of dreams ain't no flaky pop-psychology trend—it's a phenomenon celebrated throughout history by cultures as diverse as the ancient Hebrews, Egyptians, and Chinese, and is referenced in most religious texts. The ancient Greeks, for example, believed that the god of medicine Asclepius (he of the famous caduceus staff adorned with a pair of coiled snakes, still used today to symbolize the medical profession) would visit anyone who came for a nap in his temples. If he didn't miraculously cure what ailed them, he would prescribe certain herbs, practices, or healing exercises. And shamanism, perhaps the oldest spiritual system on this planet that's still alive and kicking today, uses dreams to help diagnose and cure both physical and psychological illnesses.

And then there's the Mack Daddy of all things dreamy in our modern Western culture (and an inspiration for this very piece of writing): Carl Jung. Genius Swiss psychotherapist extraordinaire, Jung analyzed thousands of patients and over 80,000 dreams in his career, and concluded that many dreams aren't merely mental masturbation, our synapses randomly firing back and forth just to give the brain something to do while we snooze. Oh no no no. In fact, Jung found that the imagery in his patients' dreams often facilitated psychological, emotional, spiritual, *and* physical healing, and that *every* dream has potential to teach us something about ourselves. And after 80,000 dreams, he should know.

In other words, dream healing has been *around,* baby. Cosmic catnaps with benefits have been happening since time immemorial. (By the way, as you probably know, there are thousands of Jungian analysts still practicing today, all over the world, as well as countless shamans.) The psychological and mystical aspects of the dream world are far more involved and dense than I can possibly go into here, but for now, just know that you have VIP access to myriad healing possibilities every time you shut your eyes and open your mind.

Let's Get This Pajama Party Started

Some specifics on how to start interpreting your dreams:

1. First and foremost: Keep a journal and pen next to your bed. And write the suckers down, first thing in the morning or even when you awaken in the middle of the night with a dream fresh in your mind. Write in present tense: "I'm running down the beach and my first-grade teacher is chasing me with a Vidal Sassoon curling iron." Note all the random images, in the order you remember them, without editing or letting logic get in the way. Don't like writing in the middle of the night? Get a cheap digital voice recorder and record your thoughts. Listen later and *then* write 'em down.

2. Once you've transcribed your dreams, start picking out and underlining the specific ingredients that seem to strike you or that might indicate a pattern: people, places, colors, sounds, clothes, body gestures, movements, and so on.

3. Next to each ingredient (consider listing the ingredients on another page), write down any and all personal (direct) associations and feelings you have about these elements

and images. How do they speak to you, both literally and metaphorically?

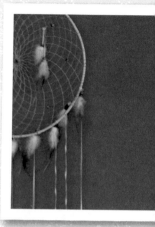

Note that dreams are notorious for weird puns. Take a dream in which your sister keeps shoving her new lipstick in your face when you're about to say something cutting and unnecessary to your mother. Your unconscious may be suggesting that you should keep your *lips sticking* together—in other words, shut it concerning this issue with your mother.

4. As you go about your day, try to be aware of any cultural significance those themes and symbols might have, any similarities within religion, psychology, mythology, fairy tales, science, and so on. Always seeing dogs, or cars, or certain trees, or green bananas in your dreams? Do a bit of research. You'd be surprised how well dream images Google. One Crazy Sexy example: the butterfly—a universal symbol for transformation, metamorphosis, rebirth, flight. Butterflies are common in dreams, and monarch butterflies in particular, despite their apparent fragility, possess incredible strength and continually astound scientists with their amazing abilities to travel immense distances to annual breeding grounds, survive all sorts of violent weather, triumph over their natural enemies, and brighten every environment.

5. You can also use what's called *active* imagining, in which you meditate or concentrate on a specific dream image you've encountered

that seems to really resonate. Allow your imagination to take off and see what turns up. Go ahead, free-associate. Write that info down, too.

6. Following a particularly vivid dream, think about what happened in the past few days. Any events stand out? Phone conversations? TV show themes that might have sparked something? A strange encounter on the bus? How might these events have triggered you?

Don't worry about making sense of your random crazy dreams, or about getting in touch with their potential healing aspects right away. Interpreting dreams is like exercising an under-developed muscle: It's only through practice and patience that the ability gets stronger. Also, our inner healer can be very persistent. Often, if we don't understand what a certain dream means, another dream hinting at the same information but in an entirely different way will show up, and then another, until one morning we scream "Eureka! I finally freaking get it!" and can move on to the next dream. (By the way, if you actually scream "Eureka," call your grandmother. She loved that word back in 1925. You'll probably say something more like "Holy shit!" after your first dream revelation. Or maybe that's just me.) Persistence is key. Keep track of your dreams for a month, and I can virtually guarantee that patterns will begin to emerge, new insights will wave hello, meanings will shift and develop.

But, But . . . I Don't Remember a Freakin' Thing!

Everyone dreams. I know you might disagree, because sometimes you can't remember a single fuzzy detail about your unconscious romps and are therefore convinced you didn't dream at all, but it's just not true (and countless studies prove it). So here are a few more tips to help you recall your dreams more vividly:

- Before you hit the hay, say to yourself, with conviction, "I will remember my dreams tonight."

- Write your dreams down *immediately* after you wake up, while you're still groggy, before you leave the salty confines of your bed to go to the bathroom, make coffee, check your e-mail, or walk your dog. Studies have shown that it only takes five minutes after the end of a dream for us to forget 50 percent of the content; ten minutes later, we've forgotten 90 percent. (The theory goes that all your dream loss is due to early-morning motor movements, as the conscious brain takes over and wipes recent subconscious activity clean.) Half an hour after you wake up, you might be convinced you didn't dream at all, when in fact you simply forgot the whole thing.

- Some believe that taking a small dose of vitamin B6 (proven to help mental clarity) helps with dream recall.

- Avoid jarring alarms in the morning, which will only hasten the quick, violent erasing of your subconscious memory. Try a natural-light alarm clock, or one of those "nature sounds" things, or a Now & Zen bell-chime alarm. Keep it gentle to keep the dreams intact as long as possible.

Strut Your Stuff

Last but not least, you need to walk your dream's talk, act on the information you receive from your inner healer. If, after you study your dream journal and feel more confident as a reader of its symbols and signs, your dreams are hinting that your current love relationship is out of balance or dysfunctional, it's usually not enough to simply say "Huh, isn't that interesting," and then just continue on in the same unhealthy way. If you're willing to look beneath your covers and be totally honest with yourself, most often the information you receive from your dreams isn't *completely* shocking. Deep down, you know there are some appropriate and timely steps you need to take to remedy the situation. So take them.

The more you become familiar with your inner universe, the more you will come to trust its guidance. After all, it's *you*—a fuzzier, stranger, but definitely wiser aspect of you—and you always have your best interests at heart. Of course, not all dream revelations require action. They might be suggesting more subtle changes, like allowing yourself to relax, release, let go, stop trying so hard to control every aspect of your life, heal your illness, always "fix" yourself.

Ultimately, all dream work is about learning to accept ourselves—the healthy parts *and* the unhealthy parts, the light and the dark, the divine and the demon, the peace and the pain, the clarity and the chaos—so we begin to recognize, on a heart level, that we're already perfect just as we are. When we reject no part of our self, when we embrace our all, we become a making of love, a superheroine, a Crazy Sexy Cowgirl, someone who can offer healing to everyone she meets. And that's not just an airy-fairy dream, my friends, but our essential reality.

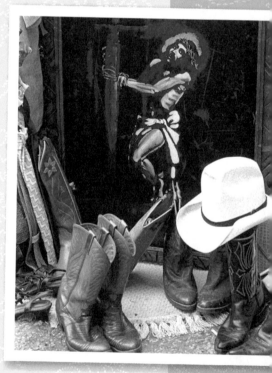

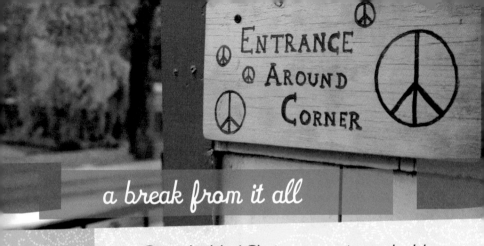

a break from it all

Happy birthday! That's correct, it's your birthday right now. Enough cancer crap. This is your day and you deserve a prezzie. For crying out loud, you've been through a heck of a lot, and if you've finished this book then you've been through a lot more. Go on a holiday in the Riviera. Even if it's just for a long weekend, change your environment and recharge your batteries on a soul vacation. If you can't afford it or don't feel well enough to voyage too far from home, treat yourself to a more low-key getaway: an overnight at a friend's house; a day trip or a long walk on an open road. Even spending an afternoon not talking about cancer can give you a healthy break. Mental vacations are just as powerful. Take this advice very seriously.

IF YOU DON'T SCHEDULE FREE TIME, YOU WILL NEGOTIATE YOURSELF OUT OF IT.

If you can't afford or don't feel well enough to take an extended vacation far from home, treat yourself to a more low-key getaway: a day trip antiquing or a long walk on a dusty open road. Even spending an afternoon just lying on a soft blanket in a pretty meadow can do wonders for the soul. What's the saying? "Sometimes you have to leave home to find it."

Spin your globe and let your finger land where it may. **Plan to travel at least once a year**—better once a season. Take cool pix, try new eats, make memories.

WRITE DOWN THE FIRST 3 PLACES THAT COME TO MIND AND THEN PLOT IT OUT.

Save your pennies so that you can live a little.

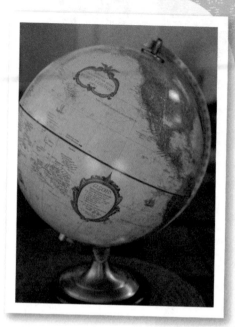

....

....

....

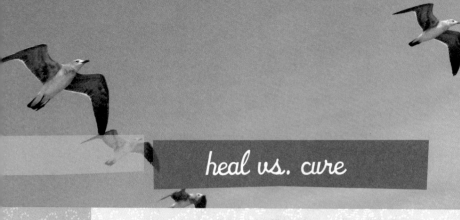

heal vs. cure

How do we define healthy? It's pretty safe to say that we no longer live in a culture where the majority of its people are disease-free. I know a lot of truly healthy people who live with cancer. Some of these people are far healthier than the average citizen. Just because an area in your body is struggling doesn't mean the entire system is broken. Everyone wants the journey to be "over," to "get their lives back." Well, if you're deeply committed to making the changes outlined in this book then what life are you going back to? You've outgrown that old paradigm. Remission? Cure? Those are wonderfully tricky words that can get us in a lot of trouble if we're living solely to hear them.

One of the first questions people ask when they find out everything I'm involved in is "Did you beat cancer? Are you in remission yet?" Yet? Oh, the pressure! At first that dreaded question took the wind out of my sails. It felt invasive and nosy, as if I were being quizzed on my net worth or, worse, my weight. But on a deeper level, I was just ashamed to admit that I hadn't kicked it yet.

- **Remission:** No signs of cancer left in your body.

- **Cured:** After five years of remission, you are considered cured.

If neither of these terms applies to you, don't fret—create your own! I used to bang my head against the wall trying to come up with ways to explain the cancer I have to people.

As hard as I tried, I was never successful. They'd scratch their heads and give me that confused what's-gonna-happen-to-you look. But as soon as I invented the term *progression-free remission*—lazy and (thankfully) unproductive tumors that just hang out like warts—they got it. Deep sigh! *Progression-free remission* was a necessary coping tool. I had the big C, which = CANCER. Now I have the little c, which = chronic. I don't think of my tumors as deadly invaders that *must* get the hell out of Dodge; I see them as a part of me that has wandered off, is confused, needs some loving, and is ready for health. It took me a long time to get to cancer (not that I created it), and healing will take an equal load of soul-maturing patience. When you embrace this lifestyle, you may expect instant changes, better scans, tumors to dissolve, and a Macy's Thanksgiving Day parade to be thrown in your honor—I did. Guess what? All those wonderful things may happen. If they do, mazel tov.

On the flip side ('cause *ka-ching* has a twin brother named *ka-splat*) you may not see one change in the cancer. It may even grow. Naturally, this will be discouraging. But let me remind you once again of the bigger picture in this *brilliant* health mosaic. You will see other ailments dissolve, you will feel empowered, you will feel like you're stepping up to the green plate of life, you will watch your relationships change, you will trim the fat and cut the deadweight, you will get closer to your God and begin to see that you have a direct line for a chat any ol' time, and you *will* heal. You may not be cured, but you will heal.

Healing, true healing is a remembering. We get out of our own way and let the love in. We move, acknowledge, accept, and revolt. We fill our bodies with the fuel (physical, mental, and spiritual) needed to shake off the darkness. No disease can thrive when we are at ease. So my goal is to carve that path, create my owner's manual and do unto others, as I would want done to me. There is only one way to really do that: Dismantle the present culture.

Nothing is guaranteed. If I could guarantee that juice and a positive attitude would "cure" you I'd be a zillionaire.

I can't. What I can promise is that you will grow and create peace. Quality is far more important than quantity. When I stopped focusing on being cured I started healing and living in a *ginormous* way.

Sometimes we'll move like crabs in life and in cancer. Crabs get to the joint, but they skitter sideways and backward to do it. Your setbacks are part of the process—hard to imagine but true. Cancer really doesn't want to kill you. After all, you're the host. If it screws up this bash, who else is gonna buy the keg?

There is a time and a season for healing. Don't compare yourself with others. Anxiety, stress, and frustration do not cure cancer. Trust and believe that your healing has begun in a BIG way. Take your mind off the cure and raise the bar on your standard of living. If you have doubts, remember to act "as if." Sometimes we need to listen more than we speak, because the signs are all around us.

WHAT CANCER TERM WORKS FOR YOU?

If you may never be in remission, can you make peace with "chronic" and get on with your life?

Before we end, I gotta take a poll. Did you buy this book because you were given a sell by/use by date? Did you relapse and, like Cher, are on yet another farewell tour? Did your doctor suggest that you get your affairs in order; make a nice list of things you'd like to do before you pass? Well, when that happened to me, I gave everyone the bird and I got myself a nice mortgage! Your future isn't a luxury. There are no crystal balls, and magic carpets are just too hard to clean, so stop wasting time and start having fun! Cancer or not, we all know what it's like to long for something. Most of us spend the better part of our twenties and thirties longing for Mr. or Ms. Right and the perfect job. Once we nab that, it's off to pining for that dream house (or apartment for you urban dwellers out there). How many times do we think of our lives as really starting when "this" happens? Why does it take a challenge to our survival for us to give ourselves permission to really live? Why don't we accept the gift of life as our birthright? You are an extremely creative person. (I know because I've been secretly reading your journal— just kidding!) Set yourself up for the future that you want. This is very different from living in the future. One is a day dream, the other is a plan.

Bye for Now

They say that an apple a day keeps the doctor away. Well, I think lemons work better. For one, they are highly alkalizing. But more importantly, this lovely little citrus reminds us to take lemons and make *champagne*. Rave it up! Plan a yearly party and invite your friends over to celebrate the new and improved you. Don't forget to serve hors d'oeuvres that encourage health. And above all, wear body glitter.

Penny-toss wishes for a happy and harmonious life, my friends. Thank you for going to your edge and curtsying with me. Hug yourself right now. Wrap your arms around your body and say *I love awesome-delicious me*.

CanSer Cowgirls and dudes are cut from a different cloth. We are enrolled in the highly competitive PhD program of life; we are one step away from Buddha-hood. What is this coiled cobra at the base of your spine trying to teach you? Only you will know. When we die, all we have is memories. Make lots of them. Go to India, even if it's just for a moment in your mind's eye. Travel there. Send me a postcard. Don't forget your crazy sexy mission . . .

1. Get real
2. Eat smart
3. Shake your ass
4. Live like you mean it
5. Educate yourself
6. Go quietly inward yet speak up
7. Get involved
8. Don't sweat the small stuff
9. Focus on healing vs. curing
10. Plan for a long future BUT live in the moment

Oh and one more—**MAKE JUICE NOT WAR!**

Peace & veggies,

kris

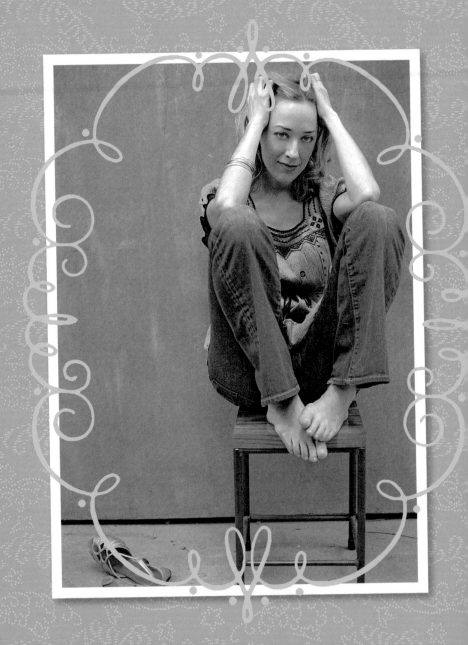